APPLIED INTELLIGENCE FOR MEDICAL IMAGE ANALYSIS

APPLIED INTELLIGENCE FOR MEDICAL IMAGE ANALYSIS

Edited by

Aarti, PhD

Raju Pal, PhD

Mukesh Saraswat, PhD

Himanshu Mittal, PhD

AAP | APPLE ACADEMIC PRESS

First edition published 2025

Apple Academic Press Inc.
1265 Goldenrod Circle, NE,
Palm Bay, FL 32905 USA

760 Laurentian Drive, Unit 19,
Burlington, ON L7N 0A4, CANADA

CRC Press
2385 NW Executive Center Drive,
Suite 320, Boca Raton FL 33431

4 Park Square, Milton Park,
Abingdon, Oxon, OX14 4RN UK

Apple Academic Press exclusively co-publishes with CRC Press, an imprint of Taylor & Francis Group, LLC

Library and Archives Canada Cataloguing in Publication

Title: Applied intelligence for medical image analysis / edited by Aarti, PhD, Raju Pal, PhD, Mukesh Saraswat, Himanshu Mittal, PhD.
Names: Aarti (Associate professor), editor. | Pal, Raju, editor. | Saraswat, Mukesh, editor. | Mittal, Himanshu, editor.
Description: First edition. | Includes bibliographical references and index.
Identifiers: Canadiana (print) 20230597378 | Canadiana (ebook) 20230597408 | ISBN 9781774914762 (hardcover) | ISBN 9781774914779 (softcover) | ISBN 9781003461852 (ebook)
Subjects: LCSH: Diagnostic imaging. | LCSH: Deep learning (Machine learning) | LCSH: Artificial intelligence—Medical applications.
Classification: LCC RC78.7.D53 A67 2024 | DDC 616.07/54—dc23

Library of Congress Cataloging-in-Publication Data

CIP data on file with US Library of Congress

ISBN: 978-1-77491-476-2 (hbk)
ISBN: 978-1-77491-477-9 (pbk)
ISBN: 978-1-00346-185-2 (ebk)

About the Editors

Aarti, PhD
Associate Professor, Lovely Professional University, India

Aarti, PhD, is working as Associate Professor at Lovely Professional University. She has more than seven years of experience in teaching. She is currently working on optimization of nature-inspired algorithms for the medical field. She is passionate about working in the area of data mining, machine learning, and optimization of learning techniques in the field of medical images and fault-tolerance. She has published more than 20 papers in the field of mining, security, and medical image analysis. She is a reviewer for many journals. She earned her PhD and MTech at Dr. B. R. Ambedkar National Institute of Technology, Jalandhar, India.

Raju Pal, PhD
Assistant Professor, Department of Computer Science and Engineering, School of Information and Communication Technology, Gautam Buddha University, Greater Noida, India

Dr. Raju Pal has more than eleven years of teaching and research experience. He is currently Assistant Professor in the department of computer science and engineering, school of information and communication technology at Gautam Buddha University, Greater Noida. He was formerly a faculty member in the Department of Computer Science and Engineering at Jaypee Institute of Information Technology, Noida, India, where he earned his doctorate degree in Medical Images Analysis. He is passionate in the area of machine learning, medical image analysis, and wireless sensor networks. He has made substantial contributions to the field of image processing and machine learning with many published research articles of high repute. He was part of the successfully completed SERB-DST (New Delhi) funded project on Histopathological Image Analysis. He is the reviewer of many international journals, including the Journal of Communications and Networks, Future Generation Computer Systems, Neural Computing and Applications, etc.

Mukesh Saraswat, PhD
Associate Professor, Jaypee Institute of Inormation Technology, Noida, UP, India

Mukesh Saraswat, PhD, has more than 18 years of teaching and research experience. He has guided two PhD students and more than 50 MTech and BTech dissertations and is presently guiding five PhD students. He has published more than 40 journal and conference papers in the area of image processing, pattern recognition, data mining, and soft computing. He is a part of the successfully completed DRDE-funded project on image analysis and is currently running two projects funded by SERB-DST (New Delhi) on histopathological image analysis and Collaborative Research Scheme (CRS), under TEQIP III (RTU-ATU) on Smile. He has been an active member of many organizing committees of various conferences and workshops. He was also a guest editor of the *International Journal of Swarm Intelligence*. He is an active member of IEEE, ACM, and CSI professional bodies. His research areas include image processing, pattern recognition, data mining, and soft computing.

Himanshu Mittal, PhD
Associate Professor, Department of Artificial Intelligence and Data Sciences, Indira Gandhi Delhi Technical University for Women, Delhi, India

Dr. Himanshu Mittal has more than eleven years of teaching and research experience. He is currently Associate Professor in the Department of Artificial Intelligence and Data Sciences at Indira Gandhi Delhi Technical University for Women, Delhi, India. He was formerly a faculty member in the Department of Computer Science and Engineering at Jaypee Institute of Information Technology, Noida, India, where he earned his doctorate degree. His interest areas include deep learning, machine learning, medical image analysis, and soft computing. He has published research publications in the field of image analysis. He is one of members of the successfully completed SERB-DST funded project on Histopathological Image Analysis. He is the reviewer of many international journals, including Future Generation Computer Systems, International Journal of Machine Learning and Cybernetics, etc.

Contents

Contributors

K. K. Anilkumar
Department of Electronics & Communication, Cochin University College of Engineering Kuttanad, Cochin, Kerala, India

Natalia Boroday
Institute for Problems of Cryobiology and Cryomedicine of the National Academy of Sciences of Ukraine, Kharkiv, Ukraine

Deepak Chawla
Department of Neonatology, Government Medical College & Hospital (GMCH), Chandigarh, India

Nischay Dhankhar
Department of Electronics and Communication, Netaji Subhas University of Technology, Delhi, India

Amira Hadj Fredj
Electronics and Micro-electronics, University of Monastir, Faculty of Sciences, Monastir, Tunisia

Bharat Garg
Thapar Institute of Engineering and Technology, Patiala, India

Nancy Girdhar
Department of Computer Science and Technology, Amity University, Noida, India

Kateryna Golubeva
Taras Shevchenko National University of Kyiv, Kyiv, Ukraine

Jaciel David Hernandez-Resendiz
Multidisciplinary Academic Unit Reynosa-Rodhe, Autonomous University of Tamaulipas, Reynosa, Tamaulipas, Mexico

Abdelwaheb Jebnouni
Electronics and Micro-electronics, University of Monastir, Faculty of Sciences, Monastir, Tunisia

S. K. Kabilesh
Jai Shriram Engineering College, Tirupur, India

Sujata Kadu
Terna Engineering College, Navi Mumbai, India

G. Kalaiarasi
Assistant Professor, Department of ACSE, Vignan Foundation for Science, Technology and Research, Andhra Pradesh

Mudassir Hasan Khan
Centre for Interdisciplinary Biomedical and Human Factors Engineering, Aligarh Muslim University, Aligarh, India

Dmitriy Klyushin
Taras Shevchenko National University of Kyiv, Kyiv, Ukraine

Edgar Tello Leal
Faculty of Engineering and Science, Autonomous University of Tamaulipas, Victoria, Tamaulipas, Mexico

Souhir Mabrouk
Higher Institute of Technological Studies of Sousse, Sousse University, Sousse, Tunisia

Prasant Mahapatra
Academy of Scientific and Innovative Research (AcSIR), Ghaziabad, India
Biomedical Application (BMA) Group, CSIR-Central Scientific Instruments Organisation (CSIR-CSIO), Chandigarh, India

Jihene Malek
Electronics and Micro-Electronics Laboratory, Monastir University, Faculty of Sciences, Monastir, Tunisia
Sousse University, Higher Institute of Applied Sciences and Technology, Sousse, Tunisia

V. J. Manoj
Department of Electronics & CommunicationCochin University College of Engineering Kuttanad, Kerala, India

Lalit Maurya
Academy of Scientific and Innovative Research (AcSIR), Ghaziabad, India; Biomedical Application (BMA) Group, CSIR-Central Scientific Instruments Organisation (CSIR-CSIO), Chandigarh, India

D. Mohanapriya
Jai Shriram Engineering College, Tirupur, India

Vatsal Nanda
Thapar Institute of Engineering and Technology, Patiala, India

Prachi Patil
Terna Engineering College, Navi Mumbai, India

Ulises Manuel Ramirez-Alcocer
Multidisciplinary Academic Unit Reynosa-Rodhe, Autonomous University of Tamaulipas, Reynosa, Tamaulipas, Mexico

Prashant Singh Rana
Thapar Institute of Engineering and Technology, Patiala, India

T. M. Sagi
Department of Medical Laboratory Technology, St. Thomas College of Allied Health Sciences, Changanacherry, Kerala, India

J. Abdul Samath
Department of Computer Science, Chikkanna Government Arts College, Tirupur, India

Mohammad Sarfraz
Member, Soft Computing Research Society, New Delhi, India

B. Saritha
Jai Shriram Engineering College, Tirupur, India

Neelofer Shaheen
Department of Electrical Engineering, Aligarh Muslim University, Aligarh, India

Priya Singh
Department of Computer Science and Technology, Amity University, Noida, India

Roop Singh
Biomedical Application (BMA) Group, CSIR-Central Scientific Instruments Organisation (CSIR-CSIO), Chandigarh, India

Amit Singhal
Department of Electronics and Communication, Netaji Subhas University of Technology, Delhi, India

Tisha Singhal
Department of Computer Science and Technology, Amity University, Noida, India

Prateek Jeet Singh Sohi
Thapar Institute of Engineering and Technology, Patiala, India

V. Sridevi
Department of Computer Science, PSG College of Arts & Science and Research Scholar of Government Arts College, Udumalpet, India

Vinayak Tiwari
Department of Electronics and Communication, Netaji Subhas University of Technology, Delhi, India

Reena Tripathi
Department of Information and Technology, Delhi Technological University, Delhi, India

Bindu Verma
Department of Information and Technology, Delhi Technological University, Delhi, India

Chan Kha Vu
Taras Shevchenko National University of Kyiv, Kyiv, Ukraine

Abbreviations

ADBIS	adaptive decision-based interpolation scheme
ADPM	anisotropic diffusion of Perona and Malik
AF	adaptive filters
AMF	adaptive mean filter
ANN	artificial neural networks
ASH	American Society of Hematology
BN	batch normalization
CDR	cup-to-disc ratio
CF	cascaded filters
CNN	convolutional neural network
DBF	decision-based filters
DL	deep learning
DLSFINR	denoising SAP noise in color images
DNN	deep neural network
DPAD	detail preserving anisotropic diffusion
DR	diabetic retinopathy
DT	decision tree
FLND	fuzzy logic noise detector
FSBMMF	fast switching-based mean median filter
HF	hybrid filter
HVS	human visual system
IBINR	interpolation-based impulse noise removal
IR	infrared
IRT	infrared thermography
ITC	infrared thermographic calorimetry
KNN	*K*-nearest neighbors
LR	logistic regression
LSTM	long short-term memory
MAC	malignancy-associated changes
MAE	mean absolute error
MAPE	mean absolute percentage error
MDBUTMF	modified decision-based unsymmetric trimmed median filter
MI	mutual information

MLP	multilayer perceptron
MRI	magnetic resonance imaging
MSE	mean square error
NB	naive Bayes
ND	noise densities
NEC	necrotizing enterocolitis
NICU	neonatal intensive care unit
OD	optical disc
PCOS	polycystic ovary syndrome
PSNR	peak signal-to-noise ratio
PSO	particle swarm optimization
ReLU	rectified linear unit
RF	random forest
RMSE	root-mean-square error
RMSLE	root-mean-square-logarithmic error
RNN	recurrent neural networks
ROI	region of interest
RR	respiration rate
SAP	salt-and-pepper
SF	switching filter
SRAD	speckle reducing anisotropic diffusion
SSIM	structure similarity metrics
SVM	support vector machine
VCDR	vertical cup-to-disc ratio
VLSI	very large-scale integration
WBCs	white blood cells
WOA	whale optimization algorithm
XGB	extreme gradient boosting

Preface

This book serves as a platform for academia, researchers, and industrial technocrats working in the medical field and related domains to contribute both theoretical and practical evaluations in research pertaining to the design and implementation of secure and sustainable computing and communication technology for the medical field. The applications are listed below:

- Security and integrity solutions for the medical field.
- Energy efficient computing algorithms for medical imaging.
- Machine learning and deep learning techniques for the medical field.
- Image processing methods for improving medical image quality.
- Analysis of radiomics.

Fundamental concepts of applied intelligence for medical image analysis are illustrated in a clear and detailed manner, with explanatory diagrams wherever necessary. All the chapters are organized and described in a simple manner to facilitate readability.

CHAPTER ORGANIZATION

Every chapter is supported by technological concepts and an illustrative analysis and solution to enlighten the readers.

This book introduces novel models to address sustainable solutions for issues related to medical image analysis.

It offers perspectives for design, development, and commissioning of intelligent applications.

It also puts forward some insights into sustainable and intelligent medical imaging techniques for the future generation.

Medical imaging includes ultrasound, computing tomography, magnetic resonance imaging, microscopy images. Medical imaging is considered as a resource for research in the medical field for scientists and engineers, clinicians, undergraduate, and graduate students.

Chapter 1 discusses the comparative study of anisotropic diffusion filters for medical image denoising.

Chapter 2 provides an extensive survey on the state-of-the-art impulsive noise removal techniques for noise medical images like MRIs, X-rays, etc.

Chapter 3 presents a comparative analysis between segmentation based on particle swarm optimization and whale optimization algorithm for brain tumor detection.

Chapter 4 discusses breast cancer screening using fractal dimension of chromatin in interphase nuclei of buccal epithelium.

Chapter 5 discusses the polycystic ovary syndrome classification based on machine learning techniques.

Chapter 6 provides a detailed review on Alzheimer's disease diagnosis methods using ensemble methods and machine learning.

Chapter 7 discusses the new strategy for the prediction of diabetic retinopathy using deep learning methods and firebase technology and discusses contactless monitoring in newborns using infrared thermography. This chapter describes and explains infrared thermography used in the monitoring of vital physiological parameters during the neonatal period.

Chapter 8 presents an analysis of medical images using machine learning techniques.

Chapter 9 provides a comparative analysis of retinal disease diagnosis using machine learning techniques.

Chapter 10 discusses a new method for automated segregation of lymphoid and myeloid blasts in acute leukemia using deep learning.

Chapter 11 evaluates four deep learning architectures (LSTM, stacked LSTM, CNN-LSTM, Encoder-Decoder LSTM) for predicting patient drug expenditures.

Chapter 12 focuses on COVID-19 diagnosis. This chapter explores classifying chest X-ray images using various classifiers, with a custom artificial neural network (ANN), achieving 95.5% accuracy.

Chapter 13 uses a deep learning approach with AlexNet. This chapter automatically categorizes cardiac arrhythmia via ECG signals, achieving over 99% accuracy, surpassing traditional methods.

Chapter 14 presents a CNN-based approach to classify mammogram images as normal, benign, or malignant, obtaining a high accuracy rate of 96.4% across multiple views, enhancing breast cancer diagnosis.

Acknowledgment

I would like to thank the colleagues of the Department of Computer Science and Engineering at the Lovely Professional University and Jaypee Institute of Information Technology for their support during the writing and maintaining of this book.

Introduction

With the advancement in technology and increased innovation over the past several decades, there has been a revolution in the analysis of medical images. Software automation has given birth to vivid intelligent technologies that can analyze and interpret medical images without human intervention. For instance, the performance demonstrated by deep learning techniques in the identification of illnesses is impressive. Additionally, the accessibility to a vast array of medical images and other forms of medical data has benefited the use of intelligence to create tailored tools for disease evaluation and suppression of emerging diseases.

Machine learning has proven to be widely accepted as one of the most powerful tools for conducting research in this domain. The platform not only uses the benchmark dataset, but also applies a certain level of intelligence for analyzing and thereby reaching a conclusion in the form of a result. This book *Applied Intelligence for Medical Image Analysis* provides free access to this reasoning and framework-building research.

SALIENT FEATURES

The scope of *Applied Intelligence for Medical Image Analysis* encompases the use of intelligent systems in industry, medical, and daily life:

- Covers the application of deep learning techniques for medical image problems.
- Covers the development of future machine learning techniques and further application of existing techniques.
- Contains chapters with literature reviews using deep learning methods for medical image analysis.
- Covers the applications of medical image applications including the diagnosis of medical images, image genomics, and brain connectomics.
- Covers the latest technologies and algorithms related to the state-of-the-art medical image analysis in assessing and diagnosing diseases.

CHAPTER 1

A Comparative Study of Anisotropic Diffusion Filters for Medical Image Denoising

AMIRA HADJ FREDJ[1], JIHENE MALEK[1,2], and SOUHIR MABROUK[2]

[1]*Electronics and Micro-Electronics Laboratory, Monastir University, Faculty of Sciences, Monastir, Tunisia*

[2]*Higher Institute of Applied Sciences and Technology, Sousse University, Sousse, Tunisia*

ABSTRACT

Noise is an important factor that can reduce the image quality and its appearance. Therefore, it must be removed while preserving the texture and the characteristics of the original image. Images can be corrupted by different types of noises and the choice of the filter depends on the use of the image and its application. In fact, selecting the appropriate denoising algorithm is closely related to the kind of noise in the image. This chapter aims to present different types of filtering algorithms based on anisotropic diffusion and applied to different types of medical images to obtain the best denoising approach. At the end, a comparative study is done using quantitative and qualitative performance evaluations.

1.1 INTRODUCTION

The most important digital image processing technique is image enhancement, which refers to the description and refinement of image

Applied Intelligence for Medical Image Analysis. Aarti, Raju Pal, Mukesh Saraswat, & Himanshu Mittal (Eds.)

characteristics such as edges or contrast so that the graphical displayed become more useful for analysis.[26,27] The image improvement is achieved using a set of techniques that seek to improve the visual appearance of an image or transform the image into a more suitable shape to be analyzed by a human or a machine. Image enhancement includes grayscale manipulations and contrast leveling, noise reduction, contour sharpening, filtering, interpolation, and amplification.[20]

Noise is an important factor that leads to a significant reduction in the quality of the image or video. This signal appears automatically in an image during the process of acquisition and transmission. In fact, noise is usually generated by electronic components in medical instrumentation; it is a random signal that is still present in many medical data, even if the electronic designs try to minimize it.[14] It may come from a source part of the image capture devices, the memory location may be defective or it may be induced due to the conditions of the capture devices such as cameras, misaligned lenses, diffusion, and other adverse conditions that may be present in the atmosphere. Its identification with eyes is very difficult so that processing algorithms are necessary for a satisfactory extraction of the useful characteristics of the images. Regardless of the type and characteristics of the noise, it is an undesirable content in the image. All medical images contain obviously some proportion of visual noise.[10] This signal gives the image a granular, snowy, or textured appearance, and it hides some information which can make diagnosis difficult for a doctor. Fundamental types of noise such as Gaussian noise, salt and pepper, speckle, and many others can be found in digital images.[9] A careful study on the different types of filters is needed to select the appropriate noise to reduce it as much as possible. Image filtering is therefore a preprocessing step essential and indispensable for many applications such as image compression, segmentation, identification, merging, object recognition, and so on.[4,22,23] The appropriate filter is chosen depending on the image characteristics, which is also related to its modality. Different linear and nonlinear filtering methods have been developed depending on the noise power or the applications for which the image is intended; each filter has different mathematical or empirical bases. Various examples of noise removal techniques have been used in medical imaging: for the study of anatomical structure and the processing of MRI, ultrasound, X-ray scanner, and endoscopy images. In the field of digital image processing, linear filtering has long been a major focus; they are easy to implement and inexpensive to calculate but not well suited to "real" images obtained from physical sensors. Indeed, most of these sensors are essentially nonlinear.

This is particularly true of the human visual system (HVS). These filters are therefore unable, for example, to eliminate impulsive noise without blurring the contours. In addition, the fast increase in the power of computing systems has made the computational complexity argument largely obsolete. This is why the development of nonlinear image processing methods has been observed. Nonlinear filtering methods are very diverse. The choice of the most efficient method for medical image denoising is very complex. It depends especially on the modality and characteristics of the image. In this work, we will establish a comprehensive study of anisotropic diffusion-filtering methods. We will test each of the filtering techniques on ultrasound, IRM, CT scan, and endoscopy images; for that, we will use in the first experiment a Gaussian noise and in the second a speckle noise. We will evaluate each algorithm and establish which filtering technique is the most appropriate for each tested medical image mode. This kind of study for such different types of medical images is very limited in the literature[21] and the comparison study in this work has proven again the complexity of the nonlinear filtering of medical images.

This chapter is organized as follows: Section 1.2 presented a qualitative study of anisotropic diffusion methods. In Section 1.3, results and discussions is given. And finally, we conclude our work.

1.2 THE NONLINEAR ANISOTROPIC DIFFUSION TECHNIQUES

The use of nonlinear filtering techniques is already important in image processing applications; it gives better results than linear filtering, removing the noise without changing the image characteristics.[6,17] However, the design and the computational implementation of the nonlinear filters are more complex. These techniques modify each pixel's value on the image according to the returned value by a nonlinear function depending on the neighboring pixels. These filters are mainly used for noise elimination and edge detection.[15] The most well-known traditional function is the median filter.[24]

There is also the wavelet transformation, which is a method of nonlinear transformation; it has a good localization property and became an important tool for image filtering.[16] In literature, several works have been devoted to the anisotropic diffusion.[1–3] With the development of graphic processor and hardware platform, various implementations of those nonlinear filters have been proposed.[8,11–13] Thus, the choice of filter depends fundamentally on the image type, the noise type, and the domain of use of the image.

1.2.1 PERONA AND MALIK FILTER

Linear spatial filtering, such as the Gaussian filtering, computes the value of a pixel by merging the weighted average values of its closest neighbors. This filtering can reduce the noise amplitude variations, but it also masks details such as lines or contours, so that the resulting images appear blurry and degraded. Perona and Malik[25] developed a method based on anisotropic diffusion called anisotropic diffusion of Perona and Malik (ADPM), a multiscale edge detection and smoothing system, which is a powerful concept in image processing. The heat diffusion equation inspired the anisotropic diffusion by introducing a diffusion function "g," that depends on the image gradient.

$$\partial u / \partial t = div\ (g\ (|\nabla u|)\nabla u) \tag{1.1}$$

where ∇ and u denotes, respectively, the gradient operator and the intensity of the image, *div* is the divergence operator, and |.| denotes the magnitude. In addition, the variable t is used to list the steps of the iterations in the discrete implementation.

1.2.2 SRAD FILTER

In the work of Yu,[28] a simplified version of Lee's filter was compared with the anisotropic diffusion filter proposed by Perona and Malik, which led to a modified anisotropic diffusion technique that they called speckle reducing anisotropic diffusion (SRAD);[28] it can be written as follows:

$$u_{i,j}^{t+\Delta t} = u_{i,j}^{t} + \frac{\Delta t}{\eta_{i,j}} div\left[c_1\left(q_{i,j}^{t}\right)\nabla u_{i,j}^{t}\right] \tag{1.2}$$

where Δt is the iteration step, c1(...) is the diffusion function given by

$$c_1(q) = \frac{1}{1+\frac{\left[q^2(x,y;t)-q_n^2(t)\right]}{\left[q_n^2(t)\left(1+q_n^2(t)\right)\right]}} \tag{1.3}$$

and $q(x,y;t)$ is the instantaneous CV, which allows separating homogeneous regions from edges in bright and dark areas; it can be considered as a discretization of

$$q = \sqrt{\frac{\frac{1}{2}\left(\frac{|\nabla u|}{u}\right)^2 - \frac{1}{16}\left(\frac{\nabla^2 u}{u}\right)^2}{\left[1 + \frac{1}{4}\left(\frac{\nabla^2 u}{u}\right)\right]^2}} \tag{1.4}$$

Here, $q_{n(t)=C_n^2}$ is the speckle scale function. In the presence of speckle noise; both the SRAD with the CV play a very important role in edge detection. To compute C_n^2, the SRAD needs to identify a homogeneous region within the processed image.

1.2.3 DPAD FILTER

In 1985, Kuan proposed a denoising method for multiplicative noise without using the linear model made by Lee.[19] The filter can be written very similar to Lee's:

$$\hat{u} = \underline{u} + k_2\left(u - \underline{u}\right) \tag{1.5}$$

with

$$k_2 = 1 - \frac{1 + \frac{1}{C_u^2}}{1 + \frac{1}{C_n^2}} \tag{1.6}$$

As mentioned above, the filter proposed by Lee is the origin and the bone of the SRAD filter.

Similar to the SRAD filter technique, Aja-Fernandez[5] has developed another anisotropic diffusion filter by merging the anisotropic diffusion with Kaun's filter rather than Lee's filter. It was named "detail preserving anisotropic diffusion" (DPAD).

The method has better performance detecting image details and reducing noise. Equation 5 can be written as

$$\hat{u} = u + \left(1 - k_2\right)\left(\underline{u} - u\right). \tag{1.7}$$

Following a similar approach to that in the section above, and if we call $(C_2 = (C_u(x,t) = (1 - k_2)$, the expression of the DPAD filter can be written as follows:

$$u_{i,j}^{t+\Delta t} = u_{i,j}^{t} + \frac{\Delta t}{\eta_{i,j}} div\left[C_2\left(C_u\left(i,j;t\right)\right)\nabla u_{i,j}^{t}\right] \tag{1.8}$$

1.2.4 OSRAD FILTER

Until now, the anisotropic diffusion definition is closely related with scattering which is a scalar function changing with the location in the image. As discussed above, the Perona and Malik diffusion limit the image smoothing near the pixels with a high-gradient amplitude (edge pixels). Near an edge, the diffusion is very low, so the noise smoothing near the edge is also low. To solve this problem, diffusion functions using matrix instead of scalars have been proposed, where anisotropic diffusion allows different diffusions in separate directions related to the local geometry of the image structures. Thus, both sides diffusion of an edge can be avoided, and in the same time, diffusion along the edge can be allowed. As a result, the edge will not be smoothed neither removed during the filtering process. Let F be the flow of the diffusion matrix which is written as follows:

$$F = div(D\nabla u) \tag{1.9}$$

where D is a positive-defined symmetric matrix adapted to the image local structure, which can be written in terms of its eigenvectors v_1 and v_2 and its eigenvalues λ_1 and λ_2 as follows:

$$D = \left(v_1 \ \ v_2\right)\left(\lambda_1 \, 0 \, 0 \, \lambda_2\right)\left(v_1^T \ v_2^T\right) \tag{1.10}$$

and the gradient vector is written as

$$\nabla u = u_{v1}.v_1 + u_{v2}.v_2. \tag{1.11}$$

In his work, Karl,[18] used a 2D base (v_1^*, v_2^*) which corresponds, respectively, to unit vectors in the gradient directions and to the minimum curvature of the smoothed version of the image, obtained convoluting the image in question with a Gaussian filter with a standard deviation σ.

This base is particularly interesting in the context of very small structures in the human body such as blood vessels, where the direction of the orthogonal axis to the gradient is held by the minimum curvature. These directions are obtained as two eigenvectors of the Hessian matrix of the smoothed image H_σ. Therefore, eigenvectors are defined as follows:

$$v_1^* \parallel \nabla_{u_\sigma} \tag{1.12}$$

$$v_2^* \perp \nabla_{u_\sigma} \tag{1.13}$$

where ∇_{u_σ} is the gradient of the image convoluted by a Gaussian filter with a standard deviation of σ, v_2^* gives an approximation on the direction of the vessels, and v_1^* its orthogonal. In addition, the diffusion function used by Karl is based on the eigenvalues of Eq. 10, it is associated with each vector of the base combining the first-order derivative of intensity in that direction. This method replaces the traditional norm of the smoothed gradient. In addition, the diffusion can be decomposed in each direction of the orthogonal base as a sum of diffusions and the divergence operator can be explicitly written as

$$div(F) = div\left(\sum_{i=0}^{2} \varphi_i\left(u_{v_i}^*\right).\ v_i^*\right) = \sum_{i=0}^{2} div\left(\varphi_i\left(u_{v_i}^*\right).\ v_i^*\right) \tag{1.14}$$

where u_{vi}^* and φ_i indicate the first-order derivative of intensity in the v_i direction and the ith diffusion function, respectively. In addition, φ_i is chosen as one of the diffusivity functions of the traditional nonhomogeneous isotropic diffusion equation, which is dependent on the intensity first-order derivative in that direction, such as $\varphi_1\left(u_{v_1}^*\right) = u_{v_1}^* e^{-\left(\frac{u_{v_1}^*}{k}\right)^2}$ and $\varphi_2\left(u_{v_2}^*\right) = \alpha \cdot u_{v_2}^*$ with $0 < \alpha < 1$ being only a diffusion function to allow smoothing in the v_2^* direction.

1.3 RESULTS AND DISCUSSIONS

1.3.1 IMAGES CORRUPTED WITH GAUSSIAN NOISE

In medical imaging, techniques aiming to noise removal have become an essential practice for the study of various anatomical structures and the processing of MRI, ultrasound, X-ray scanner, and endoscopy images. Depending on the characteristics of the image, which also depends on its modality, the appropriate filter is chosen. The following are performed and verified with MATLAB, using a PC equipped with an Intel(R) Core (TM) i7-4510U CPU 2.60 GHz.

In this experiment, we have added an additive Gaussian noise of density 10% into the different medical images. The probability density function p of a Gaussian random variable z is given by[7]

$$P_G(z) = \frac{1}{\sigma\sqrt{2\pi}} exp^{-\frac{(z-\mu)^2}{2\sigma^2}} \quad (1.15)$$

where σ and μ are, respectively, the standard deviation and the mean value, z represents the gray level.

We have evaluated the performance of each filter by measuring the PSNR metric to identify for each medical image types, the adequate filter, and we have compared the PSNR results between different modalities of images.

In this section, we have tested the different anisotropic diffusion methods using different medical images with the parameters present in Table 1.1.

TABLE 1.1 Parameters of Different Filters.

Method	K	σ	Δ_T	η_X	tang	Iter
PMAD	30	–	0.05	–	–	70
SRAD	–	–	0.02	4 DN	–	40
DPAD	–	–	0.12	5 × 5	–	100
OSRAD	–	–	0.125	–	0.15	100

Figures 1.1–1.4 present the results of different filters and Table 1.2 show the PSNR measures for each one. The first test is done using ultrasound renal image. Since renal artery ultrasound is an examination that studies the morphology (shape) and permeability of the renal arteries which is used to detect abnormalities in blood vessels. It detects and quantifies the importance and location of any obstruction, narrowing, dilation (aneurysm), or compression of the kidney arteries. Then, having a clear and filtered image is very important to achieve such observation. Therefore, a comparative study was carried out on a renal medical image of size 256 × 256 pixels. The simulation results are shown in Figure 1.1.

It can be seen from Figure 1.1(b) and (c) that the noise level cannot be efficiently reduced and the edges of the image are not well preserved. On the other hand, with the OSRAD method shown in Figure 1.1(e), the details are well preserved; for example, for small vessels, visuality and the noise power decrease compared to other filters which allows the OSRAD technique to be embedded in medical systems.

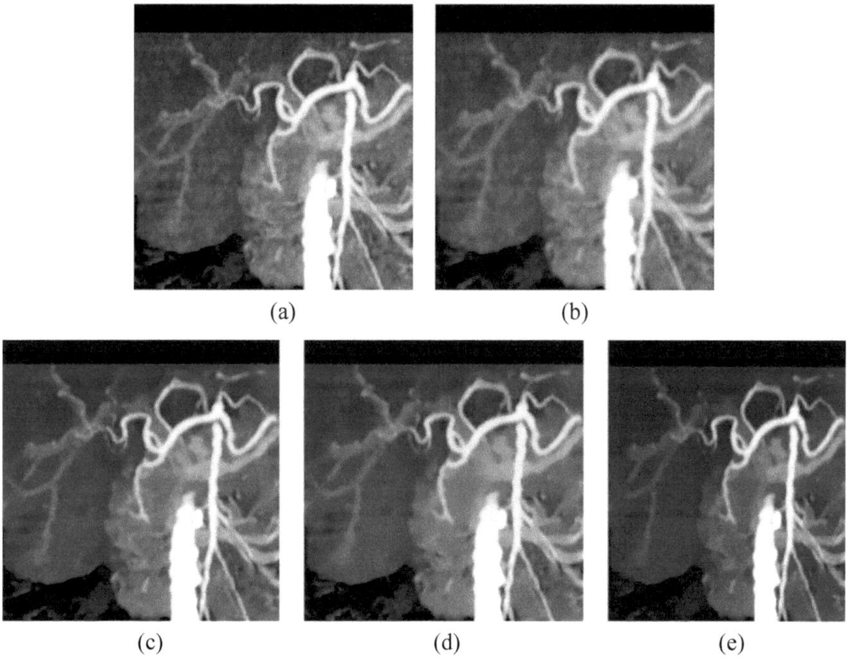

FIGURE 1.1 Results of different filters for the ultrasound renal image. (a) Original renal image; (b) PMAD filter; (c) SRAD filter; (d) DPAD filter; and (e) OSRAD filter.

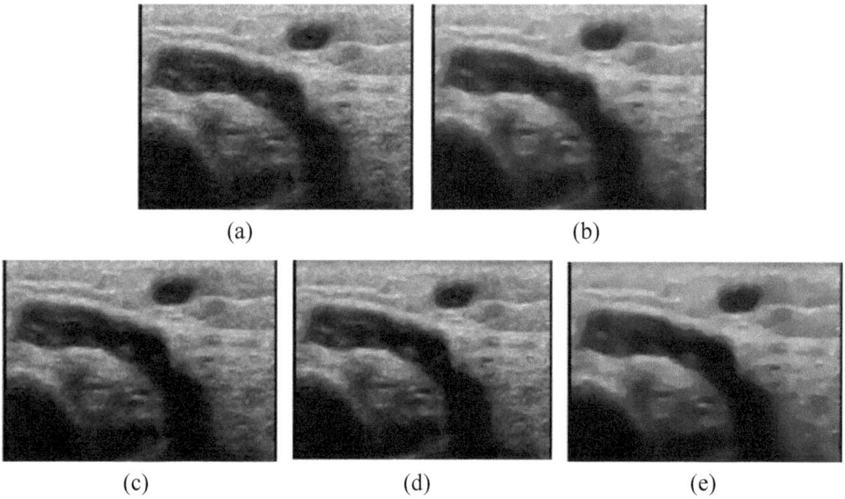

FIGURE 1.2 Results of different filters for the coronary artery image. (a) Original image of coronary; (b) PMAD filter artery; (c) SRAD filter; (d) DPAD filter; and (e) OSRAD filter.

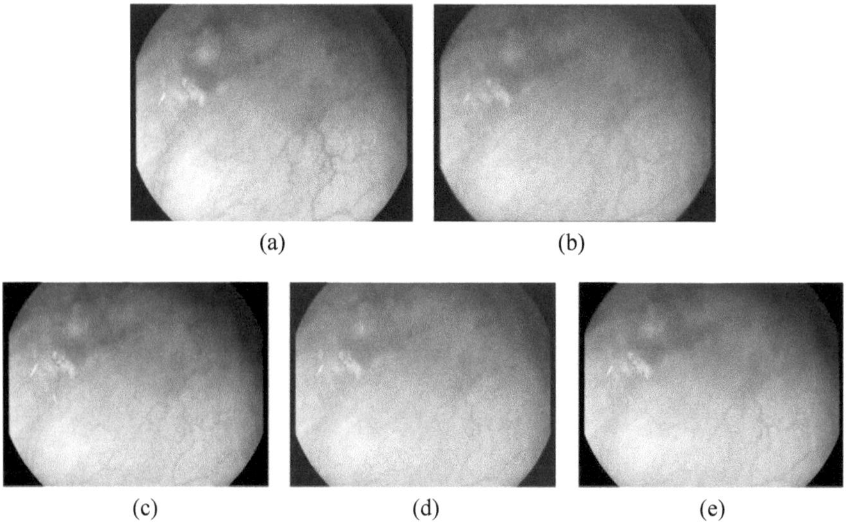

FIGURE 1.3 Results of different filters for the endoscopic image. (a) Endoscopic image; (b) PMAD filter; (c) SRAD filter; (d) DPAD filter; and (e) OSRAD filter.

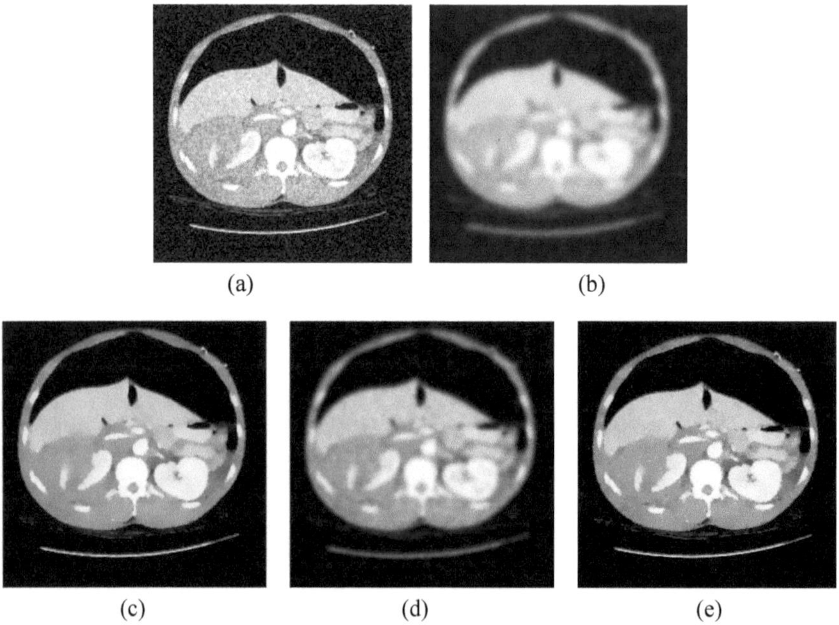

FIGURE 1.4 Results of different filters for the abdominal CT scan image. (a) Abdominal CT scan; (b) PMAD filter; (c) SRAD filter; (d) DPAD filter; and (e) OSRAD filter.

Coronary artery disease (CAD) is a complex heart disease that causes problems in the arteries that encircle and supply the heart by reducing or cutting blood flow in one or more of them.

Evaluating patients at increased risk for CAD is a very important step to save them. Different imaging modalities are used that include radiography, ultrasound, MRI fluoroscopy, multidetector CT, echocardiography, cardiac perfusion scintigraphy, and positron emission tomography.

In general, these images are affected by multiplicative noise that occurs from medical devices, which requires a preprocessing step to have a better diagnosis.

The visual evaluation of different techniques shows that the PMAD and OSRAD methods are the most efficient in terms of quality.

According to Table 1.2, the OSRAD technique is the most appropriate for filtering renal ultrasound images and abdominal images, with a PSNR of 45.80 dB and 55.97 dB, respectively. According to Figure 1.2(e), the OSRAD method preserves the different details of the image so it reduces noise in homogeneous areas and in the edges. On the other hand, the SRAD technique is the most suitable for artery coronary images as shown in the results. The PMAD and OSRAD methods were able to filter additive noise in this type of image but cannot preserve noncontrast objects.

For endoscopic imaging, the OSRAD and DPAD methods effectively reduce noise by preserving small vessels, while the PMAD method remove them and present a blurred effect with a PSNR of 18 dB.

TABLE 1.2 Comparison of Filtering Results in PSNR (dB) for Ultrasound, IRM, CT Scan, and Endoscopy with Gaussian Noise of Density 10%.

Image	SRAD	PMAD	OSRAD	DPAD
Ultrasound renal	35	25.35	45.80	35.12
IRM	42.23	34.12	30.02	22.34
Scanner X	46.94	18.88	55.97	22.46
Endoscopy	22.6	18	39.7	41.41

1.3.2 IMAGES CORRUPTED WITH SPECKLE NOISE

In this section, we have conducted the same experiences using images affected with speckle noise of density 10%. Figure 1.5 presents the filtering results of different anisotropic methods with the parameters shown in

Table 1.3. For the ultrasound image in Figure 1.5, there is a multiplicative noise content, this can add more difficulty to its removal if compared to the additive noise; in this case, the noise intensity varies with the intensity within the image. Visually, for all methods, we see that the noise is reduced in some areas of the image and not in others and the OSRAD filter is the most suitable with a PSNR of 30.39 dB (Table 1.4). For the image of a coronary artery, the noise is not well reduced but the different shape of the image is preserved. The SRAD filter is the most appropriate for denoising, this type of medical image with a PSNR of 23.26 dB. As shown in the third line of Figure 1.5, the endoscopic image is enhanced with all the anisotropic diffusion methods; therefore, the OSRAD one presents the higher value of PSNR which is equal to 36.51 dB.

For the abdominal CT scan image, the anisotropic diffusion methods are not recommended for reducing speckle noise, the shape, and the details of the image are not well preserved with an average PSNR of 21 dB.

TABLE 1.3 Simulation Parameters of Different Filters.

Method	K	σ	ΔT	η_X	tang	iter
PMAD	20	–	0.1	–	–	30
SRAD	–	–	0.19	4 DN	–	40
DPAD	–	–	0.12	3 × 3	–	40
OSRAD	–	–	0.10	–	0.15	50

TABLE 1.4 Comparison of Filtering Results in PSNR (dB) for Ultrasound, IRM, CT Scan, and Endoscopy with Speckle Noise of Density 10%.

Image	SRAD	PMAD	OSRAD	DPAD
Ultrasound renal	25.84	27.07	30.39	28.91
IRM	23.26	21.30	21.62	21.19
Scanner X	21.64	21.22	21.95	22.29
Endoscopy	28.74	32.66	36.51	32

Noise level is an important criterion to many image processing applications. For instance, the execution of an image denoising algorithm can be much damaged due to the poor noise level estimation. Table 1.5 shows the comparison in PSNR indicates with different noise densities (ND) for endoscopy image. With a high noise level, the PSNR decreases for all the filtering methods.

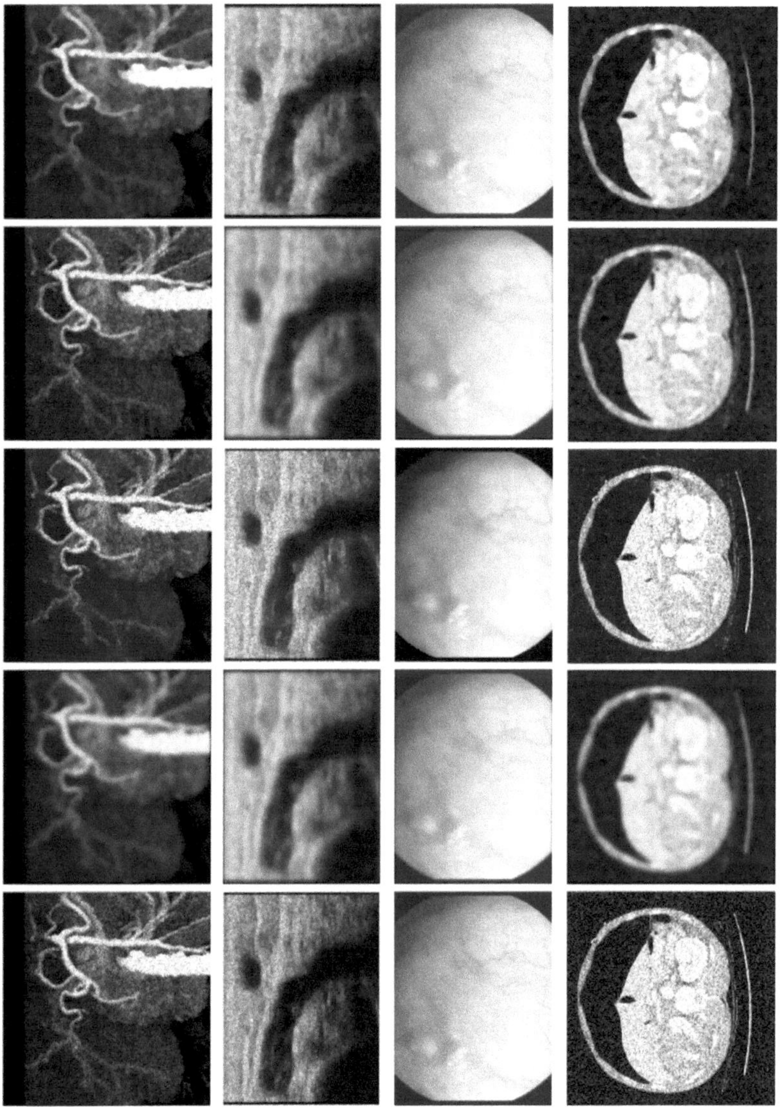

FIGURE 1.5 Results of filtering methods for different images affected by speckle noise, top to bottom: the ultrasound renal image, coronary artery image, endoscopic image, abdominal CT scan, left to right: the noisy images, PMAD, SRAD, DPAD, and OSRAD filter results.

TABLE 1.5 Comparison in PSNR (dB) with Different Level Noise for Endoscopy Image.

ND (%)	PMAD	SRAD	DPAD	OSRAD
10	32.66	28.74	32	36.51
20	31.40	28.70	32.18	35.16
30	28.46	26.25	31.03	33.90
40	25.05	22.18	26.60	31.07
50	24.84	18.77	23.50	31.07
60	22.10	18.02	21.22	28.23

1.4 CONCLUSIONS

This study introduced nonlinear filtering techniques using anisotropic diffusion for a 2D image. As it has been shown above, the objectives of this pretreatment task are to eliminate the effect of noise by preserving details and local edges between heterogeneous regions used in the image segmentation step. The most common technique of nonlinear filtering is the median filter. The value of an output pixel obtained using this latter is computed by the median of the pixels in its neighborhood. This filtering keeps the edges but causes a resolution loss by removing small details and this is not acceptable in a medical data imaging. To accomplish this task, several versions of anisotropic diffusion techniques are used, four of which have been described in this work. The main objective was to compare the performance of these four anisotropic diffusion schemes by selecting the appropriate filter for each image modality. The experiment has shown that the OSRAD method is suitable for ultrasound renal images and X-ray scanner, although the SRAD technique is adapted for MRI images and finally the endoscopic images can be filtered with the DPAD technique.

KEYWORDS

- **image processing**
- **denoising algorithms**
- **anisotropic diffusion filter**
- **medical system**

REFERENCES

1. Abdallah, M. B.; Azar, A. T.; Guedri, H.; Malek, J.; Belmabrouk, H. Noise-Estimation-Based Anisotropic Diffusion Approach for Retinal Blood Vessel Segmentation. *Neural Comput. Appl.* **2018,** *29* (8), 159–180.
2. Abdallah, M. B.; Malek, J.; Tourki, R.; Krissian, K. Restoration of Retinal Images Using Anisotropic Diffusion Like Algorithms. In *2012 International Conference on Computer Vision in Remote Sensing*; IEEE: New York, NY, 2012; pp 116–121.
3. Abdallah, M. B.; Malek, J.; Tourki, R.; Monreal, J. E.; Krissian, K. Automatic Estimation of the Noise Model in Fundus Images. In *10th International Multi-Conferences on Systems, Signals & Devices 2013 (SSD13)*; IEEE: New York, NY, 2013; pp 1–5.
4. Abidi, A.; Nouira, I.; Bedoui, M. H. Parallel Implementation on GPU for EEG Artifact Rejection by Combining Fastica and TQWT. In *2018 IEEE/ACS 15th International Conference on Computer Systems and Applications (AICCSA)*; IEEE: New York, NY, 2018; pp 1–8.
5. Aja-Fernández, S.; Alberola-López, C. On the Estimation of the Coefficient of Variation for Anisotropic Diffusion Speckle Filtering. *IEEE Trans. Image Process.* **2006,** *15* (9), 2694–2701.
6. Areshin, Y. O.; Zaikin, B.; Kotov, A.; Reshetnyak, S. Algorithm for Nonlinear Filtering of the Coordinates of a Fluctuating Object in a Bistatic Radio System. *J. Commun. Technol. Electron.* **2019,** *64* (3), 187–192.
7. Bovik, A. C. *Handbook of Image and Video Processing*; Academic Press: Cambridge, MA, 2010.
8. Fredj, A. H.; Abdallah, M. B.; Malek, J.; Azar, A. T. Fundus Image Denoising Using FPGA Hardware Architecture. *Int. J. Comput. Appl. Technol.* **2016,** *54* (1), 1–13.
9. Fredj, A. H.; Malek, J. Real Time Ultrasound Image Denoising Using NVIDIA CUDA. In *2016 2nd International Conference on Advanced Technologies for Signal and Image Processing (ATSIP)*; IEEE: New York, NY, 2016; pp 136–140.
10. Fredj, A. H.; Malek, J. GPU-Based Anisotropic Diffusion Algorithm for Video Image Denoising. *Microprocess. Microsyst.* **2017,** *53*, 190–201.
11. Fredj, A. H.; Malek, J. Performance Comparison of FPGA, GPU and CPU for an Anisotropic Diffusion Filter. *Int. J. Imaging Robot.* **2018,** *18* (3).
12. Fredj, A. H.; Malek, J.; BayBourennane, E. An Efficient FPGA Implementation of Anisotropic Diffusion Function for Medical Images. In *2018 15th International Multi-Conference on Systems, Signals & Devices (SSD)*; IEEE: New York, NY, 2018; pp 865–869.
13. Fredj, A. H.; Malek, J.; et al. Fast Oriented Anisotropic Diffusion Filter. In *2016 11th International Design & Test Symposium (IDT)*; IEEE: New York, NY, 2016; pp 308–312.
14. Gravel, P.; Beaudoin, G.; De Guise, J. A. A Method for Modeling Noise in Medical Images. *IEEE Trans. Med. Imaging* **2004,** *23* (10), 1221–1232.
15. Jain, P.; Tyagi, V. A Survey of Edge-Preserving Image Denoising Methods. *Inf. Syst. Front.* **2016,** *18* (1), 159–170.
16. Joel, T.; Sivakumar, R. An Extensive Review on Despeckling of Medical Ultrasound Images Using Various Transformation Techniques. *Appl. Acoust.* **2018,** *138*, 18–27.

17. Karnaukhov, V.; Mozerov, M. Fast Non-Local Mean Filter Algorithm Based on Recursive Calculation of Similarity Weights. *J. Commun. Technol. Electron.* **2018,** *63* (12), 1475–1477.
18. Krissian, K.; Westin, C. F.; Kikinis, R.; Vosburgh, K. G. Oriented Speckle Reducing Anisotropic Diffusion. *IEEE Trans. Image Process.* **2007,** 16(5), 1412–1424.
19. Kuan, D. T.; Sawchuk, A. A.; Strand, T. C.; Chavel, P. Adaptive Noise Smoothing Filter for Images with Signal-Dependent Noise. *IEEE Trans. Pattern Anal. Mach. Intell.* **1985,** *2*, 165–177.
20. Malek, J.; Tourki, R. Inertia-Based Vessel Centerline Extraction in Retinal Image. In *2013 International Conference on Control, Decision and Information Technologies (CoDIT)*; IEEE: New York, NY, 2013, pp 378–381.
21. Mohd Sagheer, S. V.; George, S. N. A Review on Medical Image Denoising Algorithms. *Biomed. Sign. Process. Cntrl.* **2020,** *61*, 102036. https://doi.org/10.1016/j.bspc.2020.102036. URL https://www. sciencedirect.com/science/article/pii/S1746809420301920
22. Nouira, I.; Abdallah, A. B.; Bedoui, M. H.; Dogui, M. Localisation of Epileptic Cerebral Activity Generators by 3D Spline Interpolation. In *Biosignals*, 2016; pp 340–345.
23. Nouira, I.; Ben Abdallah, A.; Layouni, S.; Bedoui, M. H.; Dogui, M. Spectral Density Variation Mapping of Cerebral Waves by Three-Dimensional Interpolation Techniques. *Int. J. Imaging Syst. Technol.* **2015,** *25* (3), 191–198.
24. Omer, A. A.; Hassan, O. I.; Ahmed, A. I.; Abdelrahman, A. Denoising CT Images Using Median Based Filters: A Review. In *2018 International Conference on Computer, Control, Electrical, and Electronics Engineering (ICCCEEE)*; IEEE: New York, NY, 2018; pp 1–6.
25. Perona, P.; Malik, J. Scale-Space and Edge Detection Using Anisotropic Diffusion. *IEEE Trans. Pattern Anal. Mach. Intell.* **1990,** *12* (7), 629–639.
26. Singh, H.; Kumar, A.; Balyan, L. A Sine-Cosine Optimizer-Based Gamma Corrected Adaptive Fractional Differential Masking for Satellite Image Enhancement. In *Harmony Search and Nature Inspired Optimization Algorithms*; Springer: Cham, 2019, pp 633–645.
27. Varatharajan, R.; Manogaran, G.; Priyan, M. K.; Sundarasekar, R. Wearable Sensor Devices for Early Detection of Alzheimer Disease Using Dynamic Time Warping Algorithm. *Cluster Comput.* **2018,** *21* (1), 681–690. DOI:10.1007/s10586-017-0977-2.
28. Yu, Y.; Acton, S. T. Speckle Reducing Anisotropic Diffusion. *IEEE Trans. Image Process.* **2002,** *11* (11), 1260–1270.

CHAPTER 2

Salt-and-Pepper Noise Removal Techniques for Medical Image Reconstruction

VATSAL NANDA, PRATEEK JEET SINGH SOHI, BHARAT GARG, and PRASHANT SINGH RANA

Thapar Institute of Engineering and Technology, Patiala, Punjab, India

ABSTRACT

This chapter provides an extensive survey on the recent denoising techniques to remove impulsive noise in medical images like MRIs and X-rays. It summarizes the progress that has been made over the years in the filters and their application involving medical image processing. Initially, different noise models are presented and then various denoising filters are discussed and compared their denoising performance in medical images. Further, their practical implications and their application are presented. This chapter also presents the mathematical expressions/flowcharts of filters for better understanding. This chapter also includes a thorough analysis of the filters by stating their strengths and weakness. Extensive comparisons are made to cover all the denoising filters and their results. The denoising quality is assessed by various quality metrics such as mean square error, peak signal-to-noise ratio, and structure similarity metrics. The time complexity is noted by noting the time taken by the particular filter for denoising. With the help of this chapter, researchers working in the image processing can quickly do their literature survey on

Applied Intelligence for Medical Image Analysis. Aarti, Raju Pal, Mukesh Saraswat, & Himanshu Mittal (Eds.)

the denoising and will get a very good comparative analysis of salt-and-pepper noise removal techniques.

2.1 INTRODUCTION

Noise is an unwanted, disruptive, unpleasant, loud sound which is disruptive to hearing. Sometimes the term noise also means signals that are random and do not carry any useful/valuable information. A special kind of noise which is totally random in nature and occurs in images is known as impulse noise. This can be seen from the lack of sharpness and preservation of structures in the image. It consists of sparse arrangement of pixels which results in the pixels to attain random values of 0 (black) and 255 (white). The general formula for calculating which pixel is corrupted and which is uncorrupted is given as follows:

$$P_{nlmg} = \begin{cases} 0 & if\ (P_{x,y} = 0 \,\|\, 255) \\ 1 & (otherwise) \end{cases} \tag{2.1}$$

where "0" represents a corrupted pixel if it has a value of 0 or 255 and "1" otherwise. The three main causes of this are fluctuations in electricity, heat, and sensor illumination levels. Such fluctuations are found to be most common during transmission of images, faulty pixels in camera, low tube current for CT, MRI, and X-ray images. This has also been a cause of concern in the medical sphere as corrupted images can result in an incorrect diagnosis putting patient's health at risk. So, various filters are introduced to reduce this impulse noise for the natural and medical images. An example of image denoising using various filters is shown in Figure 2.1. In the figure, a small part of a noisy Lena image is considered and the corresponding denoised images using various filters are demonstrated.

This chapter provides a comprehensive and an extensive summary on all those filters. Qualitative and quantitative results of multiple filters on various benchmark images (both natural and medical), at various noise densities ranging from 10% to 90%, are given in the coming sections. While doing so, we have compiled and recorded all the quantity and quality metrics of the images, namely, peak signal-to-noise ratio (PSNR), structure similarity metrics (SSIM), and mean square error (MSE), and time complexity of these filters. In the end, a compiled table gives the strengths and limitations of various filters which gives the reader perspective and discretion as to which filters among the existing ones remove the salt-and-pepper (SAP) noise efficiently and what are the limitations of some filters which could be worked upon to make them more efficient.

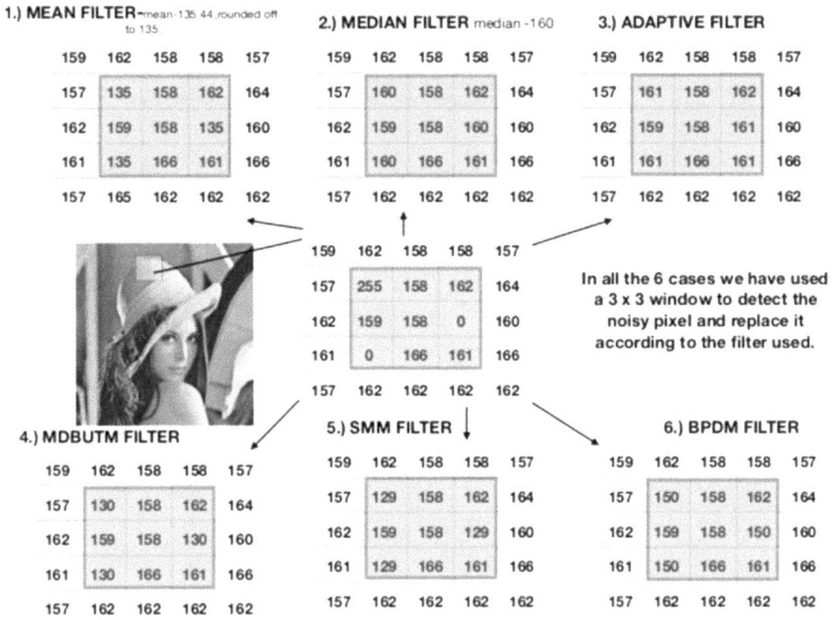

FIGURE 2.1 An illustration of image denoising via different filters.

2.2 LITERATURE REVIEW

The various state-of-the-art SAP noise removal techniques are discussed in the following subsections and are summarized in Figure 2.2.

2.2.1 LINEAR FILTERS

In linear filtering techniques, the noisy image is processed by passing it through linear functions, namely, mean, average, Gaussian, anisotropic, and improved BPDF filters, which can be referred from Figure 2.2. Various linear filters are discussed below.

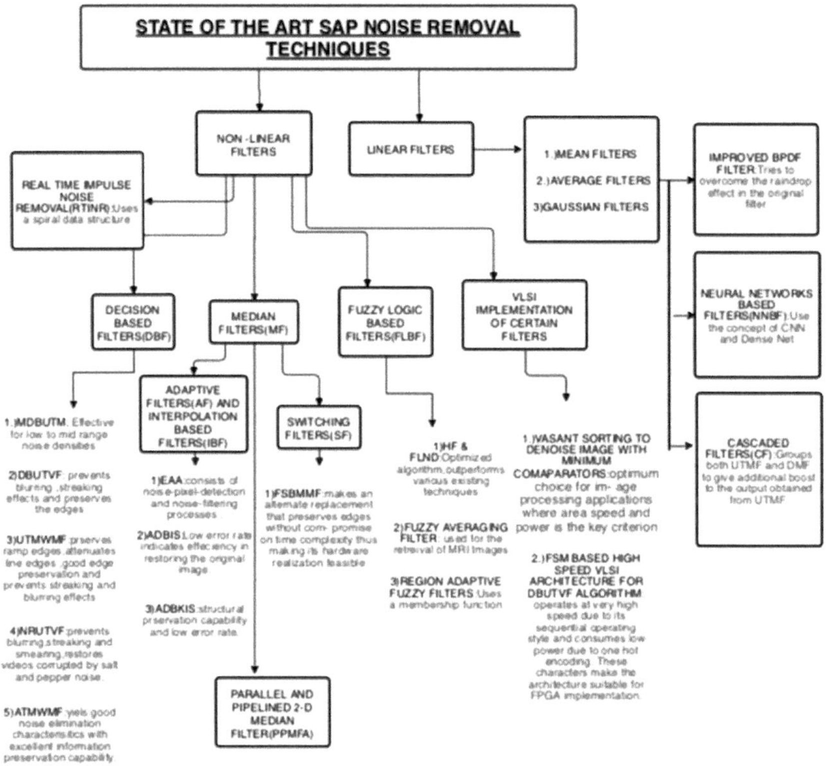

FIGURE 2.2 Flowchart for related work.

2.2.1.1 LINEAR FILTERS

A simple mean filter is a very simple filtering technique and works just fine at low noise densities. It replaces all corrupted pixels with the mean value of their corresponding neighborhood. However, its performance at higher levels of image corruption is unsatisfactory when compared to more modern filtering techniques.

2.2.2 NEURAL NETWORK-BASED FILTERS

Convolutional neural network (CNN)–based structures are used to eliminate the impulse noise. This concept is used a lot for medical image denoising. Densely connected network[1] uses the concept of dense net learning which strengthens the feature propagation. The network consists of CNN layers and batch normalization (BN) layers along with the rectified linear unit (ReLU) only. ReLU is used as the activation function in the whole architecture. BN accelerates the training procedure. The network is trained on some images from Set10 and 10 images from Set68 dataset. This architecture uses pre-activation BN which is different from the earlier deep neural network architectures. This structure is quite lightweight and has better denoising abilities than the original deep neural network algorithms.

As the above method can only be applied to SAP noise but not on Poison and Rican noise, a deep learning-based switching filter (SF) for denoising SAP noise in color images (DLSFINR)[2] was introduced which is a SF that uses a deep neural network. This network uses deep learning methods and adaptive mean filter (AMF) to detect which pixels are corrupted and which are not. The network consists of CNN layers followed by a ReLU and BN. The first layer comprises CNN and ReLU; the second and all the adjacent layers contain CNN, ReLU, and BN; and the last layer uses only convolution. This method is unique in a way as it is able to denoise colored images apart from gray-scale images. But this method is not able to detect and retain the corrupted pixels in a single stage.

Therefore, various cascaded filters (CF) are presented which are discussed in the following section.

2.2.3 NONLINEAR FILTERS

In this filtering, noisy image is processed by passing it through a nonlinear function, namely, median, decision base, and fuzzy logic-based filter. The classification of various nonlinear filters can be seen from Figure 2.2.

2.2.3.1 CASCADED FILTERS

The CF[3] uses a 3×3 fixed window over the image pixel matrix. These pixel values are placed in increasing order and it is saved in a 1D array. If the pixel values are extreme, then they are removed from the array and median of neighboring pixels is placed in the array in place of the corrupted pixels. It preserves the texture and the edges at 90% noise densities. But this method cannot be used for random-valued impulse noise removal. Therefore, an improved BPDF filter was presented which is discussed in the following section.

2.2.3.2 IMPROVED BPDF FILTER

The unique part about the BPDF technique is the way in which noisy pixels are detected. A pixel does not classify as noisy if its value is 0 or 255 but assumes all the values below 10 and above 245 as noisy.[4] The threshold value can be determined depending on the noise density (ND) levels. The size of window is increased when the noisy pixel is not found. The BPDF removed the SAP noise by considering the count of the pixels and replaces them with the median value, as has been proposed in many filters. But the BPDF filter does not perform well at high noise densities and causes raindrop effect, so the improved BPDF filter[5] was developed which uses two window sizes of 3 × 3 and 7 × 7. If there is a minimum one noisy pixel in the first window size, then median value restores the noisy pixels. Otherwise, the current window size increases to 7 × 7 and does the same procedure as it does in the 3 × 3 window.

2.2.3.3 MEDIAN FILTERS

In this kind of filtering technique, we check the center pixel of the selected. If it is corrupted, then the pixel is restored by the median of the selected window.[6] But if the pixel is not corrupted, then the window size increases. But these methods have high time complexity as the window size keeps on increasing which makes the method computationally heavy. The median filter comprises adaptive, switching, parallel, and pipelined 2D median filters (Figure 2.2), which are discussed below.

Adaptive filters and interpolation-based filters: In this category of filters, the noisy pixel is replaced by the median value of the processing window constructed around the noisy pixel.[6] Most techniques in this category use variable-size windows or use an iterative approach by making use of previously processed pixels. Form the early days of traditional simple median filter, this field has come a long way; today, we have better and more complex techniques. In Ghanekar and Pandey,[7] a 3×3 window is used which is centered at the noisy pixel of the noisy image. The noisy pixels are restored with the median of the pixels in the window. If the number of noise-free pixels (NFPs) is smaller than half of the total pixels in the window, then the size of the window is increased to 5×5. Then, the median of the NFPs is replaced with the noisy pixels in the window. Detection of impulse noise in this technique is a two-step process. First, the probable gray levels of noise are detected, and second, the noisy pixels are segregated from the noise-free ones. This filter can be applied on monochrome as well as colored images. This method has its merits and produces desired results over various benchmarks. However, its usage of larger window sizes for restoration of segments with relatively low-density results in a blurred output.

The AMFs[8] also work the same as median filters; they overcome the drawbacks of the standard median filter. But the major drawback is that if the median of the window is also an extreme value, then the size of window is also increased which again takes a lot of computation time, hence a larger time complexity.

Interpolation-based impulse noise removal (IBINR) is a class performance-oriented technique that performs exceedingly well on various benchmarks while making a compromise on computational complexity. The other drawback that these filters suffer from is that their noise detection mechanism is primitive in nature as it results in a lot of false alarms. This has led to research into the development of more precise noise detection methods which are then coupled with interpolation-based techniques for better and more effective noise removal. However, to gain a complete understanding of these filtering techniques, we must first start from the basic IBINR filtering mechanism. The idea behind this technique is to use a fixed-size window for the replacement of noisy pixel values. All neighborhood pixels are assigned weights based on their Gaussian distance from the noisy pixel. These weighted values are then used to calculate a weighted sum that is used as a replacement for the noisy pixel. If there are no NFP within window, the corrupted pixel is restored by the value having the highest count in the selected window.

Due to the fixed size window usage in IBINR, the filters' time complexity is less but this advantage comes at the cost of its restoration ability at higher ND. To avoid this problem, an adaptive decision-based interpolation scheme (ADBIS) was introduced. This method uses the concept of adaptive window size by increasing the window dimensions based on the number of NFPs. If the number of NFPs is more than three, then the same process of the weighted average is performed as seen in IBINR. However, if the selected window has only two, one, or zero original pixels, then the window size is increased by two, four, and six, respectively. The filter is summarized in the equation given below as

$$P(x,y) = Weighted\_Avg(W_{n\times n})$$

where

$$n = \begin{cases} n; & if\,(length\,(W_{nxn}) >= n) \\ n+2; & if\,(length\,(W_{nxn}) == 2) \\ n+4; & if\,(length\,(W_{nxn}) == 1) \\ n+6; & if\,(length\,(W_{nxn}) == 0) \end{cases}$$

where W stands for the window size and n stands for the number of NFPs and how the window size changes according to their values.

The above methods do not perform well at high noise densities which give the blur effect. To combat this issue, an adaptive decision-based Kriging in terpolation algorithm[9] was introduced which goes a few steps further after calculating the Euclidean distances and the number of NFPs in the window. All the weighted distances are stored in a matrix and added row-wise. Then, these values are divided by twice the number of NFPs in the current window. After this, the uncorrupted pixels are multiplied with the weights calculated above and then this value is divided by the sum of the weights. This is how a noisy pixel value is replaced by the interpolated value. The rule for changing the window size remains the same as defined by ADBIS.

Due to the faulty noise detection which can be seen from the previous filters, an SAP removal using adaptive radial basis function interpolation[10] detected the impulse noise by the rank-ordered logarithmic difference function. It is basically a logarithmic function whose value "0"/"1" determines pixels as noisy/noise-free, respectively. If the current pixel to be processed is NFPs, its value is retained. But if the current pixel to be processed is noisy and all pixels in window are noisy, then the window size is increased by 2 and the mean of the new window is used to replace the value of the noisy pixel. Therefore, various SFs are presented which are discussed in the following section.

Switching Filters: The filters use a switching process for their output, for noise detection, correction, or both. The fast switching-based mean median filter (FSBMMF)[5] overcomes the streaking effects as shown in DBA filter and the poor noise removal capability as shown by the modified decision-based unsymmetric trimmed median filter (MDBUTMF). This filter preserves edges and does not have a high time complexity. The filter is summarized in the equation as given below:

$$P(x,y)=\begin{cases} medianW(3x3); & if(X_{min}<medianW_{3x3}<X_{max}) \\ X_{i,j-1;} & if(i==1\,||\,j==N)) \\ X_{i-1,j;} & if(i==1\,||\,i==N)) \\ median\,W(5x5); & (otherwise) \end{cases} \tag{2.2}$$

where W stands for the window size.

As these methods require very high accuracy and precision, the classification of noise and NFPs goes wrong sometimes. Therefore, parallel architectures and pipelined architectures of the 2D median filter are presented which is discussed in the following section.

Parallel and pipelined 2D median filter architecture: This method is robust at impulse noise removal and its distribution in various parts of the image.[11] The value of output pixel is determined by taking 8 pixels and a 3 × 3 moving window. For 4 pixels of the input image, the first three rows are considered. The first four columns capture three-row vectors, with respect to these three rows and each vector contains four pixels. Every row vector contains a set of 4–8 bit pixels forming a 32-bit word. Due to this, the method has a relatively low time complexity. But its optimized versions can be effectively utilized in the processing of real-time images. Therefore, various decision-based filters (DBF) are presented which are discussed in the following section.

2.2.3.4 DECISION-BASED FILTERS

In these methods, the median of selected window replaces the noisy pixels. Various DBF were proposed as discussed below.

Modified Decision-Based Unsymmetric Trimmed Median Filter: In this technique, the corrupted pixels are restored by the median of the NFPs presented in the 3 × 3 window constructed across them.[12] If NFPs are not found in the given window, then the corrupted value is replaced by the mean values of all the pixels of the window. The filter is summarized in the equation given below as

$$P(x,y) = \begin{cases} median(W_{i,j})\ (if\ length(W_{i,j})! = 0) \\ mean(W_{i,j})(Otherwise) \end{cases} \tag{2.3}$$

where W stands for the window size and $P(x, y)$ stands for the noisy pixel being processed which will either have a value 0 or 255.

As the MDBUTMF could not preserve the edges and lead to their smudging, the decision-based unsymmetrical trimmed variant filter, the decision-based neighborhood referred unsymmetrical trimmed variants filter (NRUTVF) to remove of high-density SAP noise,[13] method was introduced which uses the same method as MDBUTMF to perceive the impulse noise but replaces the noisy value in different ways. If the top, bottom, left, and right pixels with respect to the noisy pixel are also noisy, then the output is the mean of all four values. Otherwise, if the window contain are pixels as noisy, then the replaced value is the overall mean of the window. The last case is when the count of noisy pixels is less than 3, then the output is the unsymmetrical trimmed median.

As the DBNRUTVF has a high time complexity, the decision-based unsymmetrical trimmed modified winsorized mean filter (DBUTMWF)[13] method was presented which detects a pixel as noisy/non-noisy by the generalized methodology of a decision filter. Here, a fixed window of 3 × 3 is chosen wherein the matrix is sorted in a 1D array if the pixel has a noisy pixel. If all pixels in the 1D array are noisy, then the output is the mean of the entire array. Otherwise, the window is replaced by the Winsorized mean which basically replaces the smallest and largest values with the observations that are closest to it in the array and averages them. The filter is summarized in an equation as follows:

$$P(x.y) = \begin{cases} Winsorised\ Mean\ (W_{i,j}); & if\,(length(W_{i,j})! = 0) \\ mean\ (W_{i,j}); & (Otherwise) \end{cases}$$

where W stands for the window size and $P(x, y)$ stands for the noisy pixel being processed which will either have a value 0 or 255.

In DBUTMWF, the estimation varies from person to person and can generate false results, so the decision-based asymmetrically trimmed modified Winsorized median filter (ATMWMF)[14] was used DBUTMWF except the last one where only some pixels in the window are noisy. The method checks in this case that if the corrupted value is 0, then the first element of the trimmed array is duplicated, if 255 then the last element of the array is copied and if both, then both the first and last element of the trimmed array are copied. But at high noise densities, this filter might give a blur effect in the image. Other filters like DBTVF are also presented which can be seen from Figure 2.2. Therefore, various fuzzy-logic-based filters are presented which are discussed in the following section.

2.2.3.5 FUZZY-LOGIC-BASED FILTERS

Some methods utilize fuzzy-based systems. These fuzzy values are calculated by utilizing the fuzzy rules whose inputs are local features that extract information from the neighborhood of the signal value to be processed, that is, from the neighborhood of the corrupted pixel.

Removal of SAP noise using hybrid filter (HF) and fuzzy logic noise detector (FLND) first passed the image through the mean and adaptive median filter and then two more matrices are generated. The distance vector of these matrices is calculated to see if the pixel is corrupted or not with the help of FLND. If the pixel is still corrupted, then the median filter is again applied. As this filter is a hybrid of mean and adaptive filters (AF), then their errors might also be present here. Various filters like fuzzy averaging filter and region adaptive fuzzy filters are presented which can be referred from Figure 2.2.

Therefore, various very large-scale integration (VLSI) implementations of certain filters are presented which are discussed in the following section.

2.2.3.6 ND-BASED FILTERS

Noise density range sensitive mean-median filter is a filtering technique that takes decision based on ND to remove SAP noise. This method primarily focuses on three separate processing modes for low, medium, and high noise densities which differ in their treatment of corner pixels, boundary pixels, usage of pre-processed pixels of estimation, window size, and their usage of mean or media operation.

A new technique called a novel multilayer decision-based iterative filter uses multiple iterations to filter out noise while maintaining the finer details on the image. The filter consists of three stages. The first stage is the pre-edge filtering step. In this, the pixel is replaced only if, in 3 × 3 window, similar pixels are present in the horizontal, vertical, or diagonal directions. It is claimed that the most of the pixels restored are replaced by the original pixel because it might be the edge of the detail in the image. The next step is the combinational filtering step. The ND of the image is calculated and two copies of the image are made. Now, according to value of ND, layers are decided and the combination of mean and median is computed to replace with the corrupted pixel. Postsmoothing process is used in the end to enhance the image quality further.

2.2.3.7 VLSI IMPLEMENTATION OF CERTAIN FILTERS

VLSI combines millions of transistors in a single chip. These are able to provide better circuits for multimedia applications, embedded systems, and IOT. We can also see the implementation of VLSI circuits for certain filters because VLSI provides a target-specific outcome, for example, in medical field, wherein image sensing and acquisition is required. This also reduces the cost of implementation. Various VLSI architecture-based filters were proposed. VLSI architecture for Vasanth sorting with minimum comparators[15] uses a 3 × 3 window over the noisy image. Then, the row elements are sorted after which the column elements are sorted in an increasing order. The northeast, center, and the southwest elements are first arranged in an increasing manner after which the upper and lower elements of the semi-diagonal are arranged in increasing order. The northeast element is compared with the west and the lower one is placed at the north-east position and the higher one in the west. The same step is repeated for the east and the southwest element.

As the Vasanth sorting algorithm gives some delay due to the sorting at high noise densities, an FSM-based VLSI architecture for DBUTVF algorithm (FSM for DBUTVF)[16] is presented. It considers a fixed 3 × 3 window where the pixels of the window are arranged in the increasing order and finally calculates the unsymmetrical trimmed median and the midpoint of the pixels in the current window. If the pixel is corrupted, the count of the pixel determines their denoising strategies. If all the pixels are noisy, their values are retained in the window. If the count is greater than 3, then the noisy pixel is restored by unsymmetric trimmed median; otherwise, it is replaced by the midpoint. But both these methods demand some amount of high computational complexity.

Therefore, various real-time filters are presented which are discussed in the following section.

2.2.3.8 REAL-TIME IMPULSE NOISE REMOVAL

This model uses a spiral data structure and stores the weights of the pixels at the pixel locations in the matrix. The noisy pixel value is restored by the Euclidean distance as that was used in interpolation-based algorithms.[17] But the problem of false alarms, as detected in interpolation, might be present here. However, there are some other filters which could not be classified discretely but fall under the category of nonlinear filters which are discussed below.

2.2.3.9 TWO-STAGE FILTER FOR HIGH-DENSITY SAP DENOISING

This method has two stages where stage I reduces high-density impulse noise which is based on the value of the weak original pixels and stage II removes the low-density impulse noise which is based upon the median of the weak original pixels.[18] But the maximum repetitive pixels are quite effective than the median of the weak original pixels. It preserves the image details and structures. But this method is not applied to variable impulse noise.

Therefore, various support vector machine (SVM)-based filters are presented which are discussed in the following section.

2.2.3.10 SVM CLASSIFICATION

Impulse noise removal based on the SVM[19] detects corrupted and uncorrupted pixel values by using Equation 1. In the SVM filter, feature selection is the most important step of this filter which includes mean, minimum, maximum, and error of the central pixel from a 3×3 window. The data set is trained on the features selected. The features selected prevent the blurring effect.

As the above filter cannot be applied to the color images and they also require a new feature vector,[23] the improved multiclass SVM method (multi-SVM) uses the multiclass SVM method to remove high ND SAP noise from the color images. It follows the basic procedure like it did in the above filter and it goes a step further where it adopts AF procedure for the removal of SAP and also adopts new features along with the previous features. It effectively removes the high ND SAP noise but does not work well on the low-density impulse noise removal.

Therefore, a non-casual linear prediction-based AF is presented which is discussed in the following section.

2.2.3.11 NONCASUAL LINEAR PREDICTION–BASED ADAPTIVE FILTER

This method is based on adaptive window in which it depends on some default threshold values.[20] A subsection of 3 × 3 of the corrupt image is taken. The error is calculated using the non-casual linear prediction around a 3 × 3 kernel. If the error is greater than a fixed threshold value, then the window size is predicted and the adaptive vector median filtering is applied. After that, the back-substitution is applied to store the final denoised image. This method preserves image details and edges and the structure. But this method is not yet applied on real images.

Therefore, an iterative adaptive unsymmetric trimmed shock filter to remove high ND SAP noise is presented. It is discussed in the following section.

2.2.3.12 ITERATIVE ADAPTIVE UNSYMMETRIC TRIMMED SHOCK FILTER TO REMOVE HIGH ND SAP NOISE

This method detects that the pixels affected by the SAP noise are detected.[21] After that, without considering the noisy pixels which were detected in the previous stage, a trimmed Gaussian filter was applied on the input image. Then, the mentioned filter is applied on the output obtained at this stage after which the median filter was applied. This method denoises well at low, medium, and high-density noise but has the disadvantage of the introduction to the blur effect which disrupts the denoising process to some extent. Therefore, four-stage median-average filter is presented which is discussed in the following section.

2.2.3.13 FOUR-STAGE MEDIAN-AVERAGE FILTER TO RECOVER IMAGES FROM HIGH ND SAP NOISE

The filter calculates the median of a 3 × 3 and 5 × 5 window.[22] After this, the output is decided on the priority of the two windows and then the corrupted pixels, which were unchanged at the first stage, are calculated.

Again after this, the adaptive average filter is applied on the unchanged corrupted pixels at the first two stages. In the end, if there are any pixels that are left, they are denoised by the estimation based on the value of the changes pixels. This method preserves image details, edges, and structures and works well at high density of noise. But by the application of four filters, it can increase the complexity of these filters.

2.3 COMPARATIVE ANALYSIS

In this section, we present Table 2.1 where we have compared various techniques by listing out their strengths and limitations.

2.4 EXPERIMENTS RESULTS AND ANALYSIS

This section presents a comparative analysis on various filters with experimental results. The experiments are carried out on two types of images: natural images and medical images. The comparison is made on the basis of the denoised images on various different filters with noise densities varying from 10% to 90%. The various quality metrics considered for comparison are presented below.

$$PSNR = 10log_{10}(MAX^2/MSE) \tag{2.4}$$

Here, MAX represents the maximum possible value of the pixel (in this case, for 8 bits, the value of MAX can be 255).

$$SSIM(x,y) = \frac{(2\mu_x\mu_y + C_1)(2\sigma_{xy} + C_2)}{(\mu_x^2 + \mu_y^2 + C_1)(\sigma_x^2 + \sigma_y^2 + C_2)} \tag{2.5}$$

Here, μx and μy give the standard deviations in the x and y axes and C1 and C2 are the constants used for limiting the value of SSIM to "1."

Tables 2.2 and 2.3 compare the MSE, PSNR, and SSIM and the time complexity of these filters with ND varying from 10% to 90% of impulse.

Figures 2.3 and 2.4 give the PSNR and SSIM, respectively, of the Lena image and Figures 2.5 and 2.6 give the PSNR and SSIM, respectively, of the CHEST image. Figures 2.7 and 2.8 illustrate Lena and Chest images, respectively, reconstructed by various filters at varying ND.

TABLE 2.1 A Comparative Summary of State-of-the-Art SAP Noise Removal Techniques.

Filter	Filter Category	Strength	Limitations
PPMFA	Median Filter	Saves a lot of time and resources while conducting the experiments.	This algorithm needs to be optimised so that it can be applied to real time processing algorighms.
FSBMMF	Switching Filters	No streaking effects. Preserves edges.	Requires high accuracy and precision Faulty noise detection.
IBINR	Adaptive Filter	No complex mathematical calculations.	Fixed window size.
ADBKIA		Overcomes the fixed window size problem of the normal interpolation filter.	Faulty noise detection.
MDBUTMF	Decision filter	Good performance at high impulse.	Does not preserve edges and leads to smudging.
UTMWF		It preserves edges and structural details.	Generates false results because the corrupted pixel is replaced by estimation.
HF AND FLND	Fuzzy Filters	All the advantages of the hybrid filters are applicable here.	Similarly, the errors introduced by MF and AMF will be combined and produced in their hybrid.
	VLSI Architecture based Filters	Requires less area Low power	It does not mention anything about noisy or non-noisy pixel. So, the sorting loses its significance.
Improved BPD filters		Good Performance at high noise levels up to 99%.	The earlier BPDF filter caused the raindrop effects. These may also occur in the improved filter.
RTINR	Real Time Filter	Run parallel in CPU and GPU.	As the operates parallel in both CPU and GPU, it requires high end hardware configuration while consuming very high power, which may lead to system heating and in turn damage of the system and/or may produce inaccurate results.
NNBF	Neural Net-work Based Filter	Quite lightweight structure. A better de noising algorithm as compared to other methods.	Only applied to SAP noise but not on Rican and Poison noise.

TABLE 2.1 *(Continued)*

Filter	Filter Category	Strength	Limitations
TSFHD SAP		Good denoising performance. Preserves image details and structures.	Not applicable to variable noise, only fixed impulse noise.
SVM		less blurring effect.	Can't be applied on color pictures, can only be used for Gray images with the introduction of new feature vector.
Multi SVM		Good denoising at high density. Adopts new features of recent filters.	Does not work well for low noise densities.
NCLP		Preserves edge details and the image structure.	Not yet applied to real images.
IAUTSF		Denoises well at low, medium and high density impulse noises.	Produces blur effect which disrupts the de noising process.
FSMAF		Works at high density noises. Preserves image details and its structure.	The application of 4 filters can increase the complexity of the algorithm.
MIN-MAX		Works well at high noise densities up to 95%.	

TABLE 2.2 Quality and Quantity Metrics of Natural Images.

Metrics	Filter	NOISE DENSITIES(%)								
		10	20	30	40	50	60	70	80	90
PSNR	MEDIAN	34.26	30.94	28.42	26.71	25.31	23.66	121.97	19.75	17.09
	MDBUTM	37.53	33.67	33.31	29.48	28.15	26.66	25.38	23.85	21.59
	FSSBM	38.18	34.44	31.98	30.08	28.48	26.17	23.27	19.18	15.72
	RSIF	36.65	32.76	30.14	28.11	26.98	25.76	24.66	23.40	21.43
	PDBM	36.99	32.94	30.30	28.60	27.14	25.47	23.98	22.11	19.59
	DAME	38.18	34.42	32.01	30.10	28.91	27.40	26.07	24.58	22.44
	TVWA	37.45	34.31	32.16	30.40	29.23	28.87	27.76	24.83	23.01
SSIM	MEDIAN	0.97	0.94	0.91	0.87	0.82	0.76	0.68	0.56	0.37
	MDBUTM	0.98	0.96	0.94	0.91	0.88	0.84	0.80	0.74	0.63
	FSSBM	0.98	0.96	0.94	0.92	0.88	0.80	0.66	0.41	0.20
	RSIF	0.98	0.96	0.93	0.89	0.86	0.82	0.77	0.72	0.63
	PDBM	0.98	0.95	0.92	0.89	0.86	0.81	0.76	0.67	0.54
	DAME	0.98	0.96	0.94	0.92	0.89	0.86	0.82	0.76	0.67
	TVWA	0.98	0.96	0.95	0.92	0.90	0.87	0.83	0.77	0.69
Time Complexity	MEDIAN	0.490	0.478	0.467	0.462	0.505	0.510	0.478	0.526	0.563
	MDBUTM	1.795	1.833	1.805	1.809	1.966	1.933	1.958	1.731	1.494
	FSSBM	0.717	0.822	0.942	1.131	1.237	1.307	1.592	1.682	1.619
	RSIF	4.831	9.337	13.679	17.387	21.533	25.645	29.778	34.341	38.633
	PDBM	0.663	0.769	0.728	0.993	1.195	1.471	1.808	2.253	2.805
	DAME	2.923	2.964	3.121	3.225	3.167	3.39	2.924	2.778	2.448
	TVWA	0.492	0.518	0.472	0.528	0.495	0.485	0.478	0.506	0.515

TABLE 2.3 Quality and Quantity Metrics of Medical Images.

Metrics	Filter	NOISE DENSITIES(%)								
		10	**20**	**30**	**40**	**50**	**60**	**70**	**80**	**90**
PSNR	MEDIAN	49.80	46.01	43.70	41.70	39.77	38.29	36.25	33.40	28.31
	MDBUTM	53.35	49.39	46.66	44.80	42.91	41.45	39.84	37.98	28.55
	FSSBM	54.06	49.74	47.70	41.51	34.05	28.02	22.31	17.32	12.76
	RSIF	52.43	47.84	44.95	42.82	41.18	40.06	38.54	36.02	31.94
	PDBM	51.11	46.50	43.91	41.98	39.56	38.15	35.47	32.63	29.12
	DAME	54.05	50.26	47.71	45.67	44.04	42.55	41.05	39.14	35.10
	TVWA	53.99	50.64	48.40	46.54	44.88	43.21	41.55	39.55	37.18
SSIM	MEDIAN	0.999	0.997	0.995	0.992	0.986	0.980	0.965	0.935	0.845
	MDBUTM	0.999	0.998	0.997	0.995	0.993	0.990	0.985	0.975	0.869
	FSSBM	0.999	0.998	0.997	0.992	0.954	0.843	0.588	0.320	0.130
	RSIF	0.999	0.998	0.996	0.993	0.989	0.985	0.977	0.961	0.922
	PDBM	0.999	0.997	0.995	0.992	0.988	0.983	0.973	0.955	0.908
	DAME	0.998	0.998	0.997	0.996	0.994	0.991	0.987	0.978	0.953
	TVWA	0.999	0.998	0.998	0.996	0.995	0.992	0.988	0.979	0.959
Time Complexity	MEDIAN	0.566	0.562	0.597	0.564	0.570	0.563	0.569	0.591	0.584
	MDBUTM	2.53	2.4	2.7	2.17	2.12	2.34	1.997	1.952	1.633
	FSSBM	0.829	0.978	1.137	1.186	1.418	1.418	1.836	1.932	1.963
	RSIF	7.116	11.793	16.316	20.613	25.9	30.264	36.739	39.22	43.342
	PDBM	0.862	0.781	1.48	1.203	1.360	1.660	2.61	2.469	3.190
	DAME	3.72	3.211	3.264	3.300	3.357	3.274	3.268	3.64	2.691
	TVWA	0.554	0.566	0.570	0.548	0.574	0.600	0.583	0.596	0.599

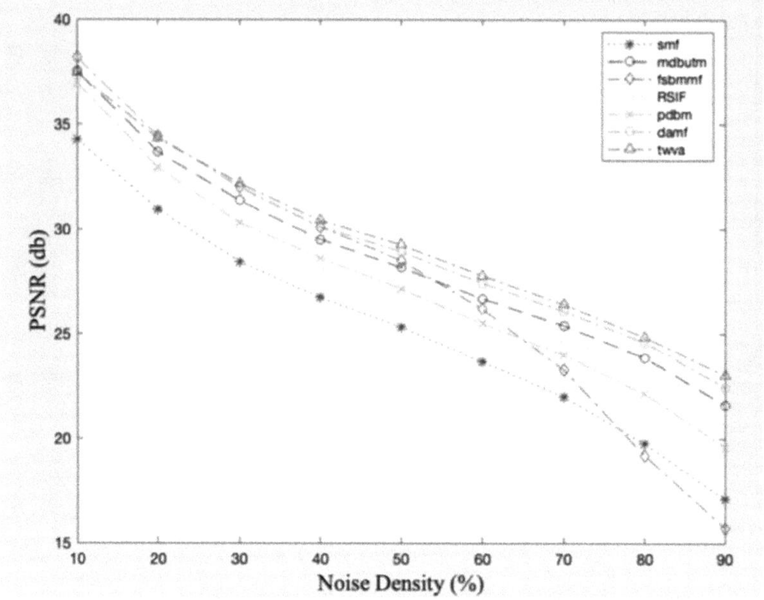

FIGURE 2.3 PSNR values for natural LENA figure.

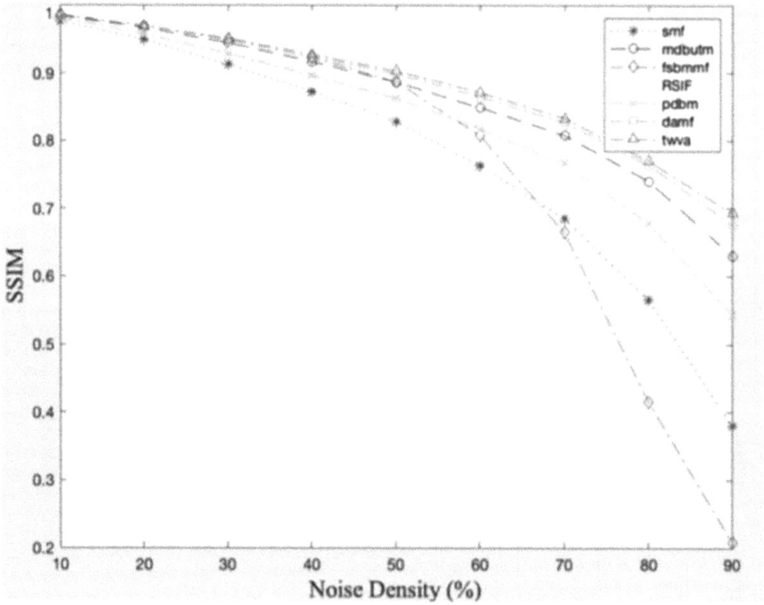

FIGURE 2.4 SSIM values for natural LENA image.

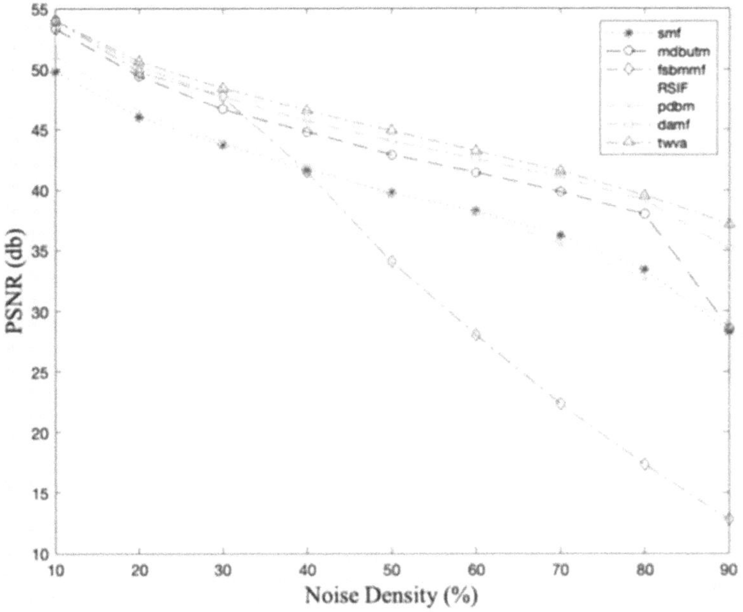

FIGURE 2.5 PSNR values for X-ray chest image.

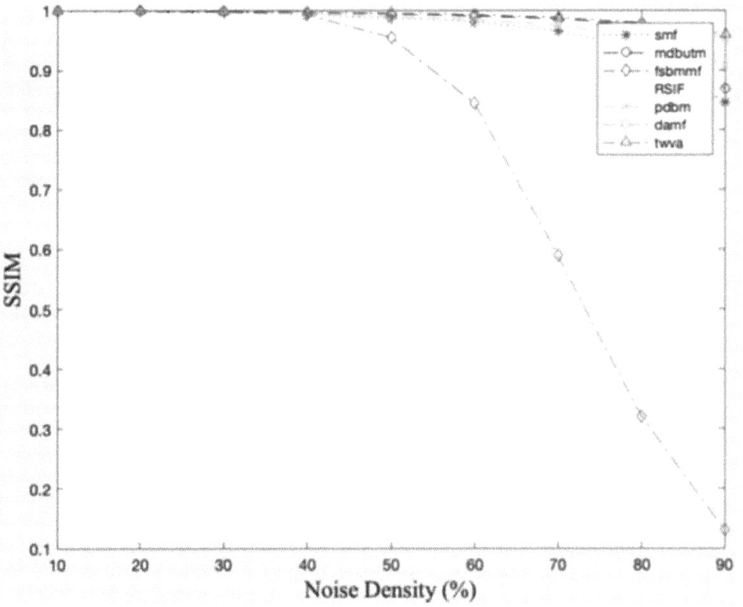

FIGURE 2.6 SSIM values for natural chest image.

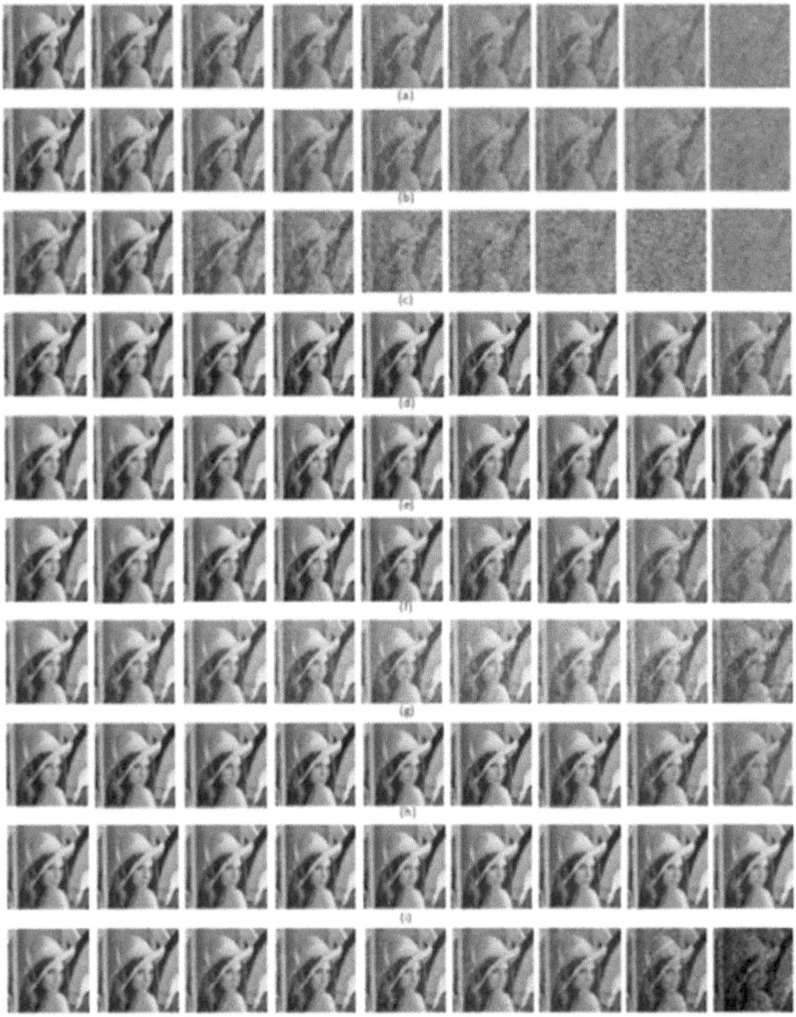

FIGURE 2.7 Comparative analysis of Lena images filter via (a) MEAN, (b) MEDIAN, (c) ADAPTIVE, (d) MDBUTMF, (e) FSBMMF, (f) DBNUTV, (g) BPDM, (h) DAMF, (i) DBIBWI, and (j) PDBM filters, respectively, applied at 10–90% noise density, column-wise (left to right).

2.5 CONCLUSION

Image denoising has become an integral part of the medical field as noisy images lead to faulty results and analysis. Image sensing, acquisition, and

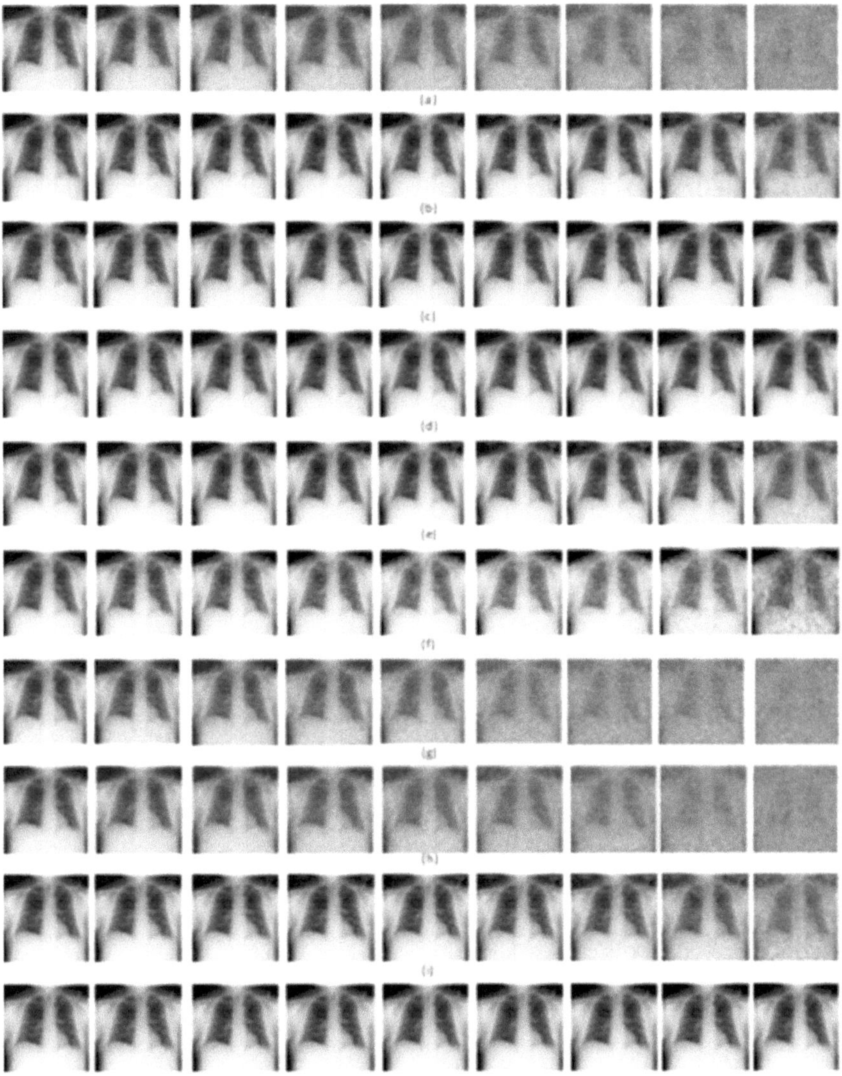

FIGURE 2.8 Comparative analysis of medical images (chest X-ray image) where (a) MEAN, (b) MEDIAN, (c) ADAPTIVE, (d) MDBUTMF, (e) FSBMMF, (f) DBNUTV, (g) BPDM, (h) DAMF, (i) DBIBWI, and (j) PDBM filters, respectively, applied at 10–90% noise density, column-wise (left to right).

recognition are also very important aspects in the medical field. This also helps in enhancing the images for a detailed analysis. This chapter gives a detailed analysis on recent impulse noise denosing techniques for medical images like MRIs, X-rays, and CT-scan. Initially, this chapter provides a detailed explanation of the filters: their algorithms, why the particular filter was used in comparison to the previous one, and what was the need to change this filter for introducing other filters. An example is illustrated for denoising noisy image using different filters. Further, a flowchart is presented to show the various methods of denoising for the ease of understanding of the reader. A comparative analysis is presented using quality metrics, namely, PSNR and SSIM, and complexity metric including execution. In the end, a table summarizing the pros and cons of the various recent filters for the ease of understanding of the reader is presented. This chapter will be helpful for those who are currently in the domain as they will be able to identify the shortcomings of various existing filters and those who are new in the field so that they can understand it easily.

KEYWORDS

- **Congo Red**
- **contour plots**
- **modified bentonite**
- **rating scale model (RSM)**

REFERENCES

1. Li, G.; Xu, X.; Zhang, M.; Liu, Q. Densely Connected Network for Impulse Noise Removal. *Pattern Anal. Appl.* **2020,** *23* (3), 1263–1275. DOI: 10.1007/s10044-020-00871-y.
2. Radlak, K.; Malinski, L.; Smolka, B. Deep Learning Based Switching Filter for Impulsive Noise Removal in Color Images. *Sensors (Basel)* **2020,** *20* (10), 2782. DOI: 10.3390/s20102782.
3. Karthik, B.; Kumar, T.; Dorairangaswamy, M.; Logashanmugam, E. Removal of High Density Salt and Pepper Noise through Modified Cascaded Filter. *Middle East J. Sci. Res.* **2014,** *20* (10), 1222–1228.
4. Erkan, U.; Gökrem, L. A New Method Based on Pixel Density in Salt and Pepper Noise Removal. *Turk. J. Elec. Eng. Comp. Sci.* **2018,** *26* (1), 162–171. DOI: 10.3906/elk-1705-256.
5. Thanh, D. N.; Thi Thanh, L.; Surya Prasath, V. B.; Erkan, U. An Improved BPDF Filter for High Density Salt and Pepper Denoising. In *2019 IEEE-RIVF International*

Conference on Computing and Communication Technologies (RIVF); IEEE: New York, NY, 2019; pp 1–5. DOI: 10.1109/RIVF.2019.8713669.
6. Brownrigg, D. R. K. The Weighted Median Filter. *Commun. A.C.M.* **1984,** *27* (8), 807–818. DOI: 10.1145/358198.358222.
7. Ghanekar, U.; Pandey, R. An Intensity Independent Fixed Valued Impulse Noise Detector for Image Restoration. *AEU Int. J. Electron. Commun.* **2014,** *68* (3), 210–215.
8. Hwang, H.; Haddad, R. A. Adaptive Median Filters: New Algorithms and Results. *IEEE Trans. Image Process.* **1995,** *4* (4), 499–502. DOI: 10.1109/83.370679.
9. Varatharajan, R.; Vasanth, K.; Gunasekaran, M.; Priyan, M.; Gao, X. Z. An Adaptive Decision Based Kriging Interpolation Algorithm for the Removal of High Density Salt and Pepper Noise in Images. *Comput. Electr. Eng.* **2018,** *70*, 447–461. DOI: 10.1016/j.compeleceng.2017.05.035.
10. Veerakumar, T.; Jagannath, R. P. K.; Subudhi, B. N.; Esakkirajan, S. Impulse Noise Removal Using Adaptive Radial Basis Function Interpolation. *Circuits Syst. Signal Process.* **2017,** *36* (3), 1192–1223. DOI: 10.1007/s00034-016-0352-1.
11. Subramaniam, J.; Kannan, R. J.; Ebenezer, D. Parallel and Pipelined 2D Median Filter Architecture. *IEEE Embedded Syst. Lett.* **2017,** *10* (3), 69–72. DOI: 10.1109/LES.2017.2771453.
12. Rajesh, P.; Kumar, E. K.; Rama, B. S.; Kishore, P. Restoration of High Density Salt and Pepper Noisy Gray & Color Videos Using MDBUTMF. *Int. J. Emerg. Technol. Adv. Eng. (IJETAE)* **2012,** *2* (9), 469–474.
13. Vasanth, K.; Jawahar Senthil Kumar, V. J. S. Decision-Based Neighborhood-Referred Unsymmetrical Trimmed Variants Filter for the Removal of High-Density Salt-and-Pepper Noise in Images and Videos. *Signal Image Video Process.* **2015,** *9* (8), 1833–1841. DOI: 10.1007/s11760-014-0665-0.
14. Christo, M. S.; Vasanth, K.; Varatharajan, R. A Decision Based Asymmetrically Trimmed Modified Winsorized Median Filter for the Removal of Salt and Pepper Noise in Images and Videos. *Multimedia Tool. Appl.* **2020,** *79* (1–2), 415–432. DOI: 10.1007/s11042-019-08124-9.
15. Vasanth, K.; Sindhu, E.; Varatharajan, R. VLSI Architecture for Vasanth Sorting to Denoise Image with Minimum Comparators. *Microprocess. Microsyst.* **2019,** *71*, 102880. DOI: 10.1016/j.micpro.2019.102880.
16. Vasanth, K.; Vadiel, M.; Kumar, S. V. G.; Ganesan, P.; Ravi, C. N.; Prasad, T. S. FSM Based High Speed VLSI Architecture for DBUTVF Algorithm. In *2019 5th International Conference on Advanced Computing & Communication Systems (ICACCS)*; IEEE: New York, NY, 2019; pp 18–22.
17. Hosseini, H.; Hessar, F.; Marvasti, F. Real-Time Impulse Noise Suppression from Images Using an Efficient Weighted-Average Filtering. *IEEE Signal Process. Lett.* **2014,** *22* (8), 1050–1054. DOI: 10.1109/LSP.2014.2381649.
18. Thanh, D. N. H.; Hai, N. H.; Prasath, V. B. S.; Hieu, L. M.; Tavares, J. M. R. S. A Two- Stage Filter or High Density Salt and Pepper Denoising. *Multimedia Tool. Appl.* **2020,** *79* (29–30), 21013–21035. DOI: 10.1007/s11042-020-08887-6.
19. Roy, A.; Laskar, R. H. Impulse Noise Removal Based on SVM Classification. In *2015 TENCON IEEE Region 10 Conference*; IEEE: New York, NY, 2015, pp 1–5. DOI: 10.1109/TENCON.2015.7373033.

20. Roy, A.; Laskar, R. H. Non-casual Linear Prediction Based Adaptive Filter for Removal of High Density Impulse Noise from Color Images. *AEU Int. J. Electron. Commun.* **2017,** *72,* 114–124. DOI: 10.1016/j.aeue.2016.12.006.
21. Veerakumar, T.; Subudhi, B. N.; Esakkirajan, S.; Pradhan, P. K. Iterative Adaptive Unsymmetric Trimmed Shock Filter for High-Density Salt-and-Pepper Noise Removal. *Circuits Syst. Signal Process.* **2019,** *38* (6), 2630–2652. DOI: 10.1007/s00034-018-0984-4.
22. Garg, B.; Arya, K. V. Four Stage Median-Average Filter for Healing High Density Salt and Pepper Noise Corrupted Images. *Multimedia Tool. Appl.* **2020,** *79* (43–44), 32305–32329. DOI: 10.1007/s11042-020-09557-3, P. 32.
23. Pal, R.; Saraswat, M.; Mittal, H. Improved Bag-of-Features Using Grey Relational Analysis for Classification of Histology Images. *Complex Intell. Syst.* **2021,** *7* (3), 1429–1443. DOI: 10.1007/s40747-021-00275-3.
24. Vijaykumar, V. R.; Santhana Mari, G. S.; Ebenezer, D. Fast Switching Based Median Mean Filter for High Density Salt and Pepper Noise Removal. *AEU Int. J. Electron. Commun.* **2014,** *68* (12), 1145–1155. DOI: 10.1016/j.aeue.2014.06.002.
25. Garg, B. Restoration of Highly Salt-and-Pepper-Noise-Corrupted Images Using Novel Adaptive Trimmed Median Filter. *Signal Image Video Process.* **2020,** *14* (8), 1555–1563. DOI: 10.1007/s11760-020-01695-3.
26. Garg, B. An Adaptive Minimum-Maximum Value-Based Weighted Median Filter for Removing High Density Salt and Pepper Noise in Medical Images. *Int. J. Ad Hoc Ubiquitous Comput.* **2020,** *35* (2), 84–95. DOI: 10.1504/IJAHUC.2020.109795.
27. Sohi, P. J. S.; Sharma, N.; Garg, B.; Arya, K. Noise Density Range Sensitive Mean Median Filter for Impulse Noise Removal. *Innovations in Computational Intelligence and Computer Vision*; Springer: Cham; pp 150–162.
28. Senthil Selvi, A.; Sukumar, R. Removal of Salt and Pepper Noise from Images Usinghybrid Filter and Fuzzy Logic Noise Detector. *Concurrency Comput. Pract. Experience* **2019,** *31* (12), e4501. DOI: 10.1002/cpe.4501.
29. Satti, P.; Sharma, N.; Garg, B. Min-Max Average Pooling Based Filter for Impulse Noise Removal. *IEEE Signal Process. Lett.* **2020,** *27,* 1475–1479. DOI: 10.1109/LSP.2020.3016868.
30. Sharma, N.; Sohi, P. J. S.; Garg, B. An Adaptive Weighted Min-Mid-Max Value Based Filter for Eliminating High Density Impulsive Noise. *Wireless Personal Communication,* 2021.
31. Sharma, N.; Sohi, P. J. S.; Garg, B.; Arya, K. A Novel Multilayer Decision Based Iterative Filter for Removal of Salt and Pepper Noise. *Multimedia Tool. Appl.* **2021,** *8,* 26531–26545.

CHAPTER 3

Comparative Analysis of PSO and WOA-Based Segmentation of Brain Tumor MRIs

REENA TRIPATHI and BINDU VERMA

Department of Information and Technology, Delhi Technological University, Delhi, India

ABSTRACT

This chapter introduces a comparative analysis between segmentations based on particle swarm optimization (PSO) and whale optimization algorithm (WOA) for brain tumor detection. This method is tailored to detect glioblastoma in MRIs. These tumors, by nature, can be anywhere in the brain and can be of any size, contrast, and shape. This motivates us to work on better detection algorithms for brain tumors. The use of a support vector machine classifier studies the efficacy of both algorithms. This contribution places itself in the literature to compare WOA and PSO in segmentation to detect brain tumors. Experimental results on the proposed approach show that WOA having 70.41% accuracy performs better than PSO with an accuracy of 66.34%.

3.1 INTRODUCTION

Segmentation of objects from images is an important prominent area in image processing and recognition of patterns that helps in many fields

Applied Intelligence for Medical Image Analysis. Aarti, Raju Pal, Mukesh Saraswat, & Himanshu Mittal (Eds.)

like medical imaging, computer vision, and many industrial applications. In the last few decades, due to advancements in image segmentation, the medical imaging field uses algorithms to detect diseases such as brain tumor detection, Parkinson's disease, Alzheimer's disease, and schizophrenia. Magnetic resonance imaging (MRI), X-rays, ultrasound, and electrocardiogram are used to analyze human disease using computer vision and pattern recognition techniques.[16]

Medical imaging takes part in detecting brain tumors, providing means to control and minimize the effects of the tumor in the patient's body. MRI is valuable data to detect the disease in the patient's body. It does not harm the patient and provides highly detailed images of the required tissue structure. It is a noninvasive technique that does not involve radiation throughout the process. When the mass of brain cells grows in an uncontrolled manner, it is known as a brain tumor. A tumor that originates in the brain itself is named a primary brain tumor. In contrast, a tumor might spread to the brain, developed in some other part of the body, and is termed a secondary brain tumor or "metastases" (https://www.aans.org/en/Patients/Neurosurgical-Conditions-and-Treatments/Brain-Tumors). Brain tumor segmentation involves dividing MRIs within different tissues such as white matter, gray matter, and cerebrospinal fluid that helps detect various diseases.

Image segmentation is a process that involves dividing the image manually or automatically into sets of regions having similar properties. Manual detection and segmentation of brain tumors are time-taking, costlier, and error-prone, and accuracy is not up to that mark. Even for experienced and professional radiologists, there can be variations in the diagnosis process. These problems can be overcome by building an automated process to detect brain tumors from MRIs efficiently. Segmenting brain tumors from MRIs can assist to make better diagnostics, predicting tumor growth rate and planning the future treatment approach. Hence, to make detection cost-effective in terms of time and efficiency, plenty of research has already been proposed for brain tumor segmentation in the literature[1–3] based on region growing, graph cut, and clustering.

Thus, inspired by automatic brain tumor segmentation to help in medical imaging, we have proposed the whale optimization algorithm (WOA) algorithm to segment a brain tumor. This chapter is a relative analysis of two nature-inspired algorithms, particle swarm optimization (PSO) and WOA. We used PSO and WOA to section the brain tumor from

MRI data and a linear support vector machine (SVM) to categorize the segmented portion into the tumor and nontumor classes. Results obtained from both algorithms and their comparative analysis show that WOA performs better than PSO. The dataset used consists of DICOM and MRI that are first converted to JPEG. Further, SVM is used to train the data and classify the tumor and nontumor.

The systematized pattern of this chapter is as follows. We talk about the related work in Section 3.2. A detailed explanation of nature-inspired algorithms has been discussed in the background study in Section 3.3. Our proposed approach is explained in Section 3.4, and a comparative analysis of PSO and WSO has been discussed in experimental results in Section 3.5. Finally, we ended in Section 3.6 with the future directive.

3.2 LITERATURE SURVEY

Brain tumor segmentation refers to the process of dividing MRIs of the brain into different tissues named cerebrospinal fluid, gray matter, and white matter. Brain tumor segmentation is a tough problem and requires a lot of research and study. Before processing for segmentation, one of the tasks is to remove unwanted artifacts and enhance the quality of images. George et al.[4] proposed a methodology to improve the quality of images for better analysis. They used histogram modeling and a median filter to detach the highest intensity noise from the images. In MRI, images of brain tumors contain the skull, which is not required for observation and segmentation. Roy et al.[5] proposed a simple skull stripping (S3) algorithm for eliminating tissues of the noncerebral area like the skull, dura, and skull from a brain MRI. Kumar et al.[1] put forward a brain tumor segmentation algorithm based upon a modified intuitionistic fuzzy *c*-means algorithm. Mekhmoukh et al.[6] presented a brain tumor segmentation algorithm that used the improved kernel possibilistic *c*-means algorithm based on PSO. They utilized spatial information from neighborhood and PSO for cluster centers and member initialization. Prastawa et al.[7] introduce a framework for detecting brain tumors from MRIs and edema.

Similarly, Corso et al.[8] introduced an efficient automatic method to detect and segment brain tumors using an integrated Bayesian model. Banerjee et al.[9] introduced a framework for 3D segmentation of brain tumors from MRI volumes based on a saliency map. Davarpanah et al.[10]

proposed a framework to segment brain tumors using symmetry spatial possibilistic FCM. It integrates spatial data and uses spatial information to compute fuzzy membership and probabilistic values.

In our chapter, we have used the WOA presented by Mirjalili et al.[11] This algorithm is stimulated by the bubble-net hunting strategy and humpback whale social behavior. The WOA is based on stimulating the finding for prey, encircling prey, and bubble-net foraging behavior of humpback whales. In our chapter, we can conclude the efficiency and drawbacks of the WOA and compare it with PSO. Multiple feature extraction techniques are proposed, such as HOG-based feature extraction[12] and geometrical feature extraction,[13] that outperform different datasets. Motivated by Verma and Choudhary,[12,13] first-order histograms and co-occurrence matrix-based features are found out and passed to SVM to segment the brain tumor.

3.3 BACKGROUND STUDY: NATURE-INSPIRED ALGORITHMS

Nature-inspired algorithms have gained popularity because of the size and complexity of many natural-world issues that are constantly increasing. These problems require the development of modes whose efficiency is judged based on their ability to find an accountable solution in an efficient time rather than an optimal solution.[17–20]

3.3.1 PARTICLE SWARM OPTIMIZATION

PSO is an optimization algorithm that iteratively improves the optimal solution. It is based on the bird's social behavior and optimization based on the population.[14] A random solution is initialized with the help of the PSO algorithm in the search space and iteratively searches for the optimal solution. Each particle is used to represent a solution. Two best values, personal best (*pbest*) and global best (*gbest*), are calculated for a particular particle in each iteration. Each particle is updated using *pbest* and *gbest* values while moving through the search space. A fitness function is used as given in Eq. 3.1.

To measure particle global optimum, closeness is used to update the global best solution and the unique desired solution of the particle. The fitness function is dependent on the optimization problem. The information of each particle is as follows:

- c_i, particle's current position.
- *pbest*$_i$, the personal best solution of particle.
- *vel*$_i$, the velocity of a particle.

If F denotes the fitness function, then each particle *pbest* value is updated using the following equation:

$$pbest_i\left(k+1\right)=\begin{cases} pbest_i\left(k\right),\ if\ F\left(c_i\left(k+1\right)\right)\geq F\left(pbest_i\left(k\right)\right) \\ c_i\left(k+1\right),\ if\ F\left(c_i\left(k+1\right)\right)<F\left(pbest_i\left(k\right)\right)\end{cases} \tag{3.1}$$

If *gbest* is the global best particle position in the search space, then

$$\begin{aligned} &gbest\in pbest_o\left(k\right),pbest_1\left(k\right),\ldots\ldots,pbest_m\left(k\right)=\min F\left(pbest_o\left(k\right)\right),\\ &F\left(pbest_1\left(k\right)\right),\ldots\ldots F(pbest_m\left(k\right)\end{aligned} \tag{3.2}$$

Equation (3.3) can be used to update the velocity of each particle:

$$\begin{aligned} &vel_i\left(k+1\right)=w.vel_i\left(k\right)+a_1.b_1(pbest_i\left(k\right)\\ &-c_i\left(k\right)+a_2\cdot b_2\cdot gbest-c_i\left(k\right))\end{aligned} \tag{3.3}$$

where a_1 and a_2 are constants of acceleration, b_1 and b_2 are random numbers ranging between 0 and 1, and w is an inertia weight. Position of particle i is updated using the following equation:

$$c_i\left(k+1\right)=c_i\left(k\right)+c_i(k+1) \tag{3.4}$$

3.3.2 WHALE OPTIMIZATION ALGORITHM

The whale is one of the fancy creatures and is famous for its hunting technique.[11] The foraging behavior of humpbacks is termed the bubble-net feeding method. This unique behavior is found only in humpback whales and can be used as a mathematical model to solve the optimization. The following sections discuss a detailed explanation of bubble-net foraging, searching for prey, and encircling prey.

3.3.2.1 ENCIRCLING PREY

Humpback whales find to locate their prey and then encircle them. The WOA algorithm supposed that the current best candidate solution is the target prey or is near to optimum. Once the best search agent is explained, the rest of the best search agent is achieved by updating the search agent position. This behavior can be explained by eq 3.5:

$$\vec{U} = \left|\vec{V} \cdot \vec{W}(k) - \vec{W}(k)\right| \tag{3.5}$$

$$\vec{W}(k+1) = \vec{W}(k) - \vec{X} \cdot \vec{U} \tag{3.6}$$

where k is the current iteration, $\vec{X}$ and $\vec{V}$ are coefficient vectors, $W*$ is the position vector of the best solution achieved yet, and $\vec{X}$ is the position vector. $W*$ is updated after each iteration if there is a better solution.

Value of $\vec{X}$ and ($\vec{V}$)can be computed using the following equations:

$$\vec{X} = 2\vec{x} \cdot \vec{m} - \vec{x} \tag{3.7}$$

$$\vec{V} = 2 \cdot \vec{m} \tag{3.8}$$

where $\vec{x}$ is linearly decreased from 2 to 0 and $\vec{m}$ is a random vector between 0 and 1.

3.3.2.2 BUBBLE-NET FORAGING

The bubble-net behavior of humpback whales can be made over by following two mathematical mechanisms:

1. Shrinking encircling mechanism: This behavior can be obtained when we decrease the value of $\vec{x}$ in eq 3.7. As the value of $\vec{x}$ decreases, the range of $\vec{X}$ also fluctuates between its value in between [-1, 1]. The new positions are then updated using:

$$\vec{W}(k+1) = \vec{W}^*(k) - \vec{X} \cdot \vec{U} \; if \; \alpha < 0.5 \tag{3.9}$$

   where α is an arbitrary number between 0 and 1.

2. Spiral updating position: In this distance between prey and whale is being calculated. Let whale at position ($W, \cdot Z$) and prey at position ($W \cdot *, \cdot Z *$), then the new position can be created by following eq 3.10.

$$\vec{W}(k+1) = \vec{U'} \cdot \beta^{bk} \cdot \cos(2\pi k) + \vec{W}^*(k) \tag{3.10}$$

   and $\vec{U'}$ = can be calculated using following eq 3.11.

$$\vec{U'} = \left|\vec{W}^*(k) - \vec{W}(k)\right| \tag{3.11}$$

Where b is a constant that defines the shape of the logarithmic spiral. Since whale uses both methods simultaneously, therefore, to model them mathematically, we use random probability α, if $\alpha < 0.5$ value of the new position is updated using eq 9 otherwise using eq 3.11.

3.3.2.3 SEARCH FOR PREY (EXPLORATION PHASE)

In case the value of $\vec{A}$ is greater than 1 or less than 1 we activate the exploration phase i.e. instead of moving toward global best we move towards the random position.

This can be given by the following mathematical model:

$$\vec{U} = \left|\vec{V} \cdot \vec{W}_{rand} - \vec{W}\right| \tag{3.12}$$

$$\vec{W}(k+1) = \vec{W}_{rand} - \vec{X} \cdot \vec{U} \tag{3.13}$$

Where, W_{rand} is an arbitrarily chosen vector from the current population. WOA algorithm starts with an arbitrary solution and searches for the global optimum solution. Thus $|A| > 1$ establishes exploration.

3.4 PROPOSED WORK

In our proposed work, we have practiced the segmentation of brain tumors from different MRIs using WOA. Then, we have used the SVM to classify the segmented portion as tumor or nontumor. WOA very first time used by us to segment the brain tumor so far. In the literature, PSO was already implemented for brain segmentation, and we did a comparative analysis with PSO in the experimental section. The flow chart presented in Figure 3.1 depicts the workflow of the proposed work. A dataset is initially collected, and basic preprocessing steps, including skull stripping, are applied to the images. The next step is the segmentation of the tumor from MRIs using PSO and WOA. For training, we have divided 70% of the data, and for testing remaining 30% of the data. A total of 13 features are selected from each segmented image and are passed to the SVM for the training of a tumor portion. The rest of the dataset is used to test the classifier that classifies the images in either tumor or nontumor class.

3.4.1 PREPROCESSING

The very first step of the implementation is preprocessing images for training which includes noise removal by local and nonlocal denoising algorithm, histogram equalization using Contrast Limited Adaptive Histogram Equalization method, and skull stripping.

3.4.1.1 SKULL STRIPPING

The skull stripping from the brain image is important as it acts as the initial step for further processing the brain images. It helps to increase the precision and reliability of the entire diagnosis process. Skull stripping involves the process of removing the skull, eyes, and scalp, called nonbrain tissues from the brain MRIs. There are two assumptions in the skull stripping: (i) the skull portion is smaller than the brain region, and (ii) secondly that the gray matter (darker in color) enclosed the white matter and cerebrospinal fluid (even darker in color) in brain MRIs. The method used at first divides the images into the brain and nonbrain regions based on the threshold value determined using the intensity value of the images. The images are converted to binary images to locate the brain surface's membrane region and calculate the threshold value. The identification of the membrane region includes the taking away of background pixels from the MRIs and computation of the mean intensity value of the region that is identified. The location of the skull is approximated utilizing the initial mean value of the whole image, and the final mean value is computed for this recognized area.

After the identification of the membrane region, the threshold value is calculated from the pixel intensity values.

The brain and the nonbrain regions are completely separated by applying the opening morphological filtering. The brain region is then obtained as the largest connected component. The region we obtained still contains holes surrounding the border of the surface of the brain because of the lesser intensity values of CSF than the calculated value of the threshold. So to get a smooth border and precise skull-stripped MRIs, a closing morphological operation is used. For denoising MRIs, median filtering is used before calculating the threshold value and the morphological operations.

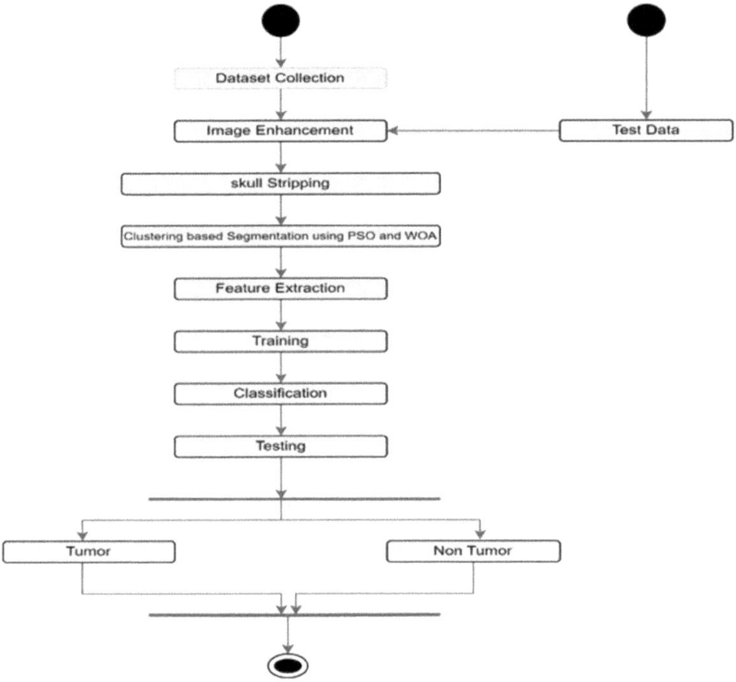

FIGURE 3.1 Flowchart of our proposed approach.

The following number of stages have been performed to find the skull stripping in the MRIs:

1. Our first step of preprocessing is to apply median filtering on input MRI data with a window size of 3×3.
2. The initial intensity value θ_i has been calculated for each input MRI.
3. We assume that the gray value of the skull is higher than θ_i, then we identify the location of each pixel in right, left, top, and bottom corners of the image from where the skull begins in the MRIs.
4. Then we create a rectangular region using the identified corner points in pixel location.
5. Then we calculate the final mean value θ_f from the created rectangular region using the pixels information.
6. By assuming that the intensity value of the skull is greater than θ_f and the intensity value of the membrane is less than θ_f, we identify the region of the brain membrane.

7. Then for the membrane, the threshold value θ is taken instead of the average intensity value.
8. Change the input MRIs into binary images with the help of the threshold θ.
9. To separate the brain and skull region, we apply the morphological operation of 13×13 opening to the binary image.
10. The largest connected component obtained is considered the brain.
11. Then to smoothen the border of the obtained region, we applied the morphological operation of 21×21 closing.

3.4.2 CLUSTERING

The next step is clustering using PSO and WSO. In both of them, clustering is done by considering the intensity value. For tumor images, we have considered four clusters for cerebrospinal fluid, white matter, grey matter, and tumor portion as these four sections have different intensity values for brain MRIs. Similarly for nontumor images, we have considered only three of them (assuming no tumor portion). For both the algorithms, the fitness function is of intracluster distance and data points are image pixel intensity values; we aim to keep similar intensity values together in the same cluster. Euclidean distance for PSO, each possible solution or particle position is set of four intensity values; intensity values of four abovementioned clusters with initial values provided randomly. Values for the max number of iterations were taken as 20, 30, 50, and 100 and it was experimentally seen that after 30, there were no changes in the fitness values. Velocity in subsequent iterations is a combined factor of inertia, cognitive factor, and social factor with an inertial weight of 0.5 and acceleration constants α_1 and α_2 as 0.4 and 0.4, respectively. The result is a set of four intensity values which are mean cluster intensity values for each abovementioned cluster. For nontumor images, this gives a set of three intensity values. Similarly, for the WOA, the max number of iterations is taken as 2.0. The images were then segmented based on cluster values and the smallest cluster is considered to be a tumor.

3.4.3 FEATURE SELECTION

Two types of features were collected:

First-order histogram features:

Mean (M), variance (V), energy (E_1), entropy (E_2), skewness (S), kurtosis (K)

Second-order gray-level co-occurrence matrix-based features:

Angular (A), second moment (SM), correlation (C), inertia (I), absolute value (AV), inverse difference (ID), entropy (E_3), maximum probability (MP)

The abovementioned features are taken for each image in the dataset and passed to the SVM as the feature vector:

$$F_v = [M, V, S, K, E_1, E_2, A, SM, C, I, AV, ID, E_3, MP] \quad (3.14)$$

3.4.4 CLASSIFICATION

SVM is considered to be the best machine learning as well as pattern recognition technique to classify the given data. SVM draws a hyperplane between two classes, and if any new data come, it calculates the margin distance and assigns it to the class with which point has the minimum distance. SVM can also be used as a multi-class classifier in which a kernel function is used to draw the hyperplane. In our proposed work, we have used linear SVM having two classes tumor and nontumor. A feature vector of 70% data has been used to train the SVM with their class labeling as a tumor and nontumor. During the testing phase, we have used 30% data, and if an unknown image is given, our approach first calculates the features and then passes them to the SVM to classify the respective class as tumor or nontumor. Experiments are performed with an SVM classifier using a quadratic kernel function. SVM classifier is trained using these features for tumor and nontumor images.

3.5 EXPERIMENTAL ANALYSIS

3.5.1 DATASET

The proposed brain tumor detection method is evaluated using MR brain tumor images from the REMBRANDT[15] database. The database contains presurgical MRIs from 130 Rembrandt patient's site datasets. The magnetic images are available in DICOM format in the database, transformed into JPEG format, and stored in a local database after processing. A total of 1000 normal and 2000 tumor MRIs are used for this work. Details of the dataset are displayed in Table 3.1. Figure 3.2 depicts the preprocessing steps in our approach. Each row from top to bottom represents original image, enhanced image, median blur image, threshold image, morphological operation, floodfill, floodfill inverse, mask, and skull stripped.

TABLE 3.1 Details of REMBRANDT[15] Dataset.

Collection statistics	
Modalities	MR
Total patients	130
Total studies	174
Total series	1483
Total number of images	110,020
Size of database	9.9

From the above-implemented procedures, it is observed that PSO provides better results as compared to WOA. While WOA gives results faster than PSO, the overall quality of the results obtained is not up to the level of results obtained from PSO. WOA relies on several probabilistic variables and the results are uncertain.

The accuracy of the PSO algorithm has been reported in Table 3.2. Similarly, the accuracy of the WOA algorithm is mentioned in Table 3.3.

TABLE 3.2 Results of PSO.

Sensitivity	97.18%
Specificity	0%
Accuracy	66.34%

TABLE 3.3 Result of WOA.

Sensitivity	99.12%
Specificity	0%
Accuracy	70.41%

Brain tumor segmentation solutions are reported in Figures 3.3 and 3.4 for tumor and nontumor data.

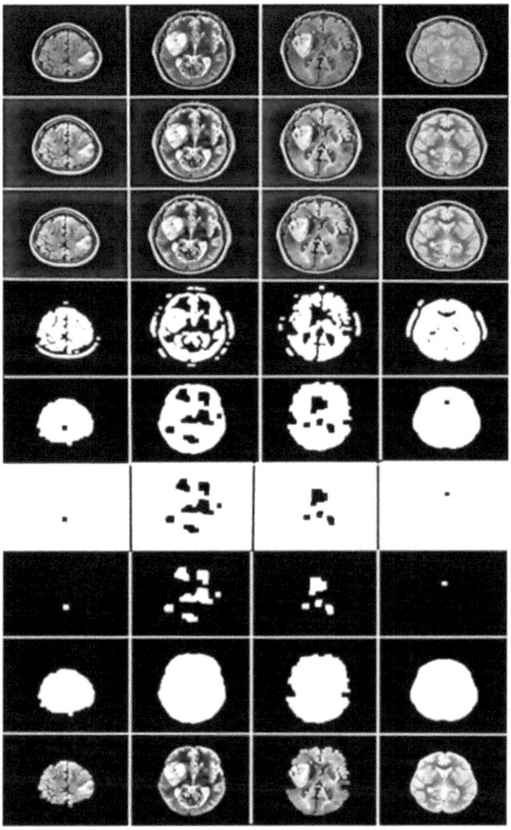

FIGURE 3.2 The preprocessing steps in our proposed approach. Each row from top to bottom represents original image, enhanced image, MedianBlur image, threshold image, morphological operation, floodfill, floodfill inverse, mask, and skull Stripped.

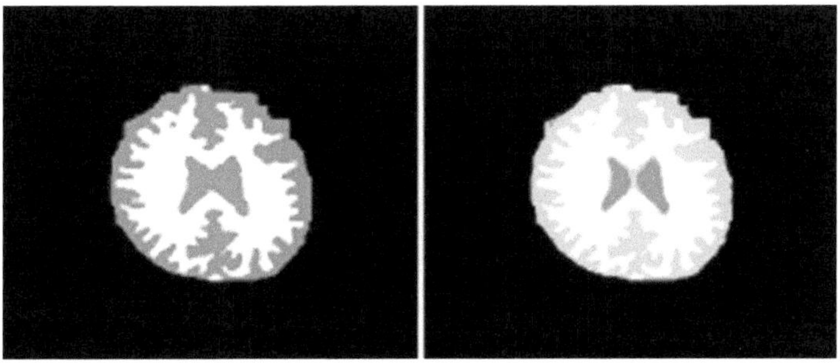

FIGURE 3.3 Segmentation of nontumor MRI with WOA and PSO.

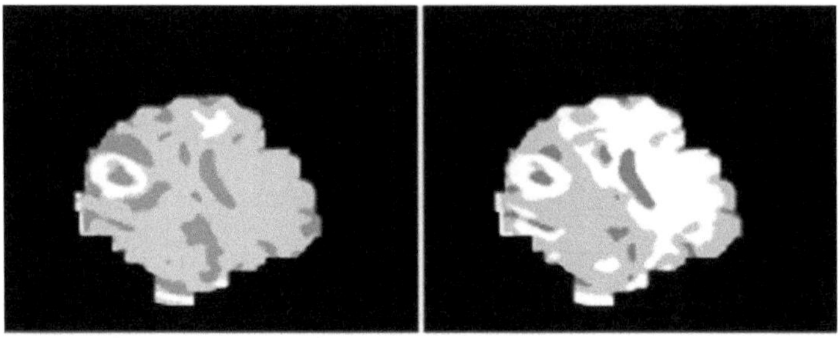

FIGURE 3.4 Segmentation of tumor MRI with WOA and PSO.

3.6 CONCLUSION

In this work, PSO and WOAs were used to segment brain tumor MRIs and SVM to train the dataset. The results achieved after the experiments show that the WOA is quicker in providing the results. Still, the overall accuracy achieved by the PSO is far superior to that obtained by WOA. The model presented in this chapter still needs to be checked for more MRIs to get a clear sense of the better algorithm between PSO and WOA for the problem of segmentation and to improve the proposed model further before it can be used in real diagnosis.

KEYWORDS

- **comparative analysis**
- **whale optimization algorithm**
- **particle swarm optimization**
- **vector machine classifier**
- **segmentation**

REFERENCES

1. Kumar, D., Verma, H., Mehra, A.; Agrawal, R. A Modified Intuitionistic Fuzzy *c*-Means Clustering Approach to Segment Human Brain MRI Image. *Multimed. Tools Appl.* **2019,** *78*, 12663–12687.

2. Nabizadeh, N.; Kubat, M. Brain Tumors Detection and Segmentation in MR Images: Gabor Wavelet vs. Statistical Features. *Comput. Electr. Eng.* **2015,** *45*, 286–301.
3. Chaira, T. A Novel Intuitionistic Fuzzy C Means Clustering Algorithm and Its Application to Medical Images. *Appl. Soft Comput.* **2011,** *11* (2), 1711–1717.
4. George, E. B.; Karnan, M. MRI Brain Image Enhancement Using Filtering Techniques. *Int. J. Comput. Sci. Eng. Technol.* **2012,** 2229–3345. https://api.semanticscholar.org/CorpusID:16283602
5. Roy, S.; Maji, P. A Simple Skull Stripping Algorithm for Brain MRI. In *Advances in Pattern Recognition (ICAPR), 2015 Eighth International Conference*; IEEE: New York, NY, 2015; pp 1–6.
6. Mekhmoukh, A.; Mokrani, K. Improved Fuzzy *c*-Means Based Particle Swarm Optimization (PSO) Initialization and Outlier Rejection with Level Set Methods for MR Brain Image Segmentation. *Comput. Methods Prog. Biomed.* **2015,** *122* (2), 266–281.
7. Prastawa, M.; Bullitt, E.; Ho, S.; Gerig, G. A Brain Tumor Segmentation Framework Based on Outlier Detection. *Med. Image Anal.* **2004,** *8* (3), 275–283.
8. Corso, J. J.; Sharon, E.; Dube, S.; El-Saden, S.; Sinha, U.; Yuille, A. Efficient Multilevel Brain Tumor Segmentation with Integrated Bayesian Model Classification. *IEEE Trans. Med. Imaging* **2008,** *27* (5), 629–640.
9. Banerjee, S.; Mitra, S.; Shankar, B. U. Automated 3D Segmentation of Brain Tumor Using Visual Saliency. *Inf. Sci.* **2018,** *424*, 337–353.
10. Davarpanah, S. H.; Liew, A. W.-C. Spatial Possibilistic Fuzzy *c*-Mean Segmentation Algorithm Integrated with Brain Mid-Sagittal Surface Information. *Int. J. Fuzzy Syst.* **2017,** *19* (2), 591–605.
11. Mirjalili, S.; Lewis, A. The Whale Optimization Algorithm. *Adv. Eng. Softw.* **2016,** *95*, 51–67.
12. Verma, B.; Choudhary, A. Framework for Dynamic Hand Gesture Recognition Using Grassmann Manifold for Intelligent Vehicles. *IET Intell. Trans. Syst.* **2018,** *12* (7), 721–729.
13. Verma, B.; Choudhary, A. Grassmann Manifold Based Dynamic Hand Gesture Recognition Using Depth Data. *Multimed. Tools Appl.* **2020,** *79* (3), 2213–2237.
14. Mohsen, F.; Hadhoud, M. M.; Moustafa, K.; Ameen, K. A New Image Segmentation Method Based on Particle Swarm Optimization. *Int. Arab. J. Inf. Technol.* **2012,** *9* (5), 487–493.
15. Scarpace, L.; Flanders, A. E.; Jain, R.; Mikkelsen, T.; Andrews, D. W. Data from REMBRANDT. *Cancer Imaging Arch.* **2015**. doi:10.7937/K9/TCIA.2015.588OZUZB.
16. Bahadure, N. B.; Ray, A. K.; Thethi, H. P. Image Analysis for MRI Based Brain Tumor Detection and Feature Extraction Using Biologically Inspired BWT and SVM. *Int. J. Biomed. Imaging* **2017,** *2017*, 9749108.
17. Pal, R.; Yadav, S.; Karnwal, R.; Aarti, EEWC: Energy Efficient Weighted Clustering Method Based on Genetic Algorithm for HWSNs. *Complex Intell. Syst.* **2020,** *6* (2), 391–400.
18. Pal, R.; Saraswat, M. A New Weighted Two-Dimensional Vector Quantisation Encoding Method in Bag-of-Features for Histopathological Image Classification. *Intell. Inf. Syst. Intell. Database Syst.* **2020,** *13* (2–4), 150–171.

19. Pandey, A. C.; Pal, R.; Kulhari, A. Unsupervised Data Classification Using Improved Biogeography Based Optimization. *Int. J. Syst. Assur. Eng. Manage.* **2018,** *9* (4), 821–829.
20. Pal, R.; Saraswat, M. Improved Biogeography-Based Optimization. *Int. J. Adv. Intell. Paradigms* **2018,** *10* (1), 1.

CHAPTER 4

Breast Cancer Screening Using Fractal Dimension of Chromatin in Interphase Nuclei of Buccal Epithelium

DMITRIY KLYUSHIN[1], KATERYNA GOLUBEVA[1], NATALIA BORODAY[2], and CHAN KHA VU[1]

[1]*Taras Shevchenko National University of Kyiv, Kyiv, Ukraine*

[2]*Institute for Problems of Cryobiology and Cryomedicine of the National Academy of Sciences of Ukraine, Kharkiv, Ukraine*

ABSTRACT

We propose new method of breast cancer diagnosis using fractal dimension of Feulgen-stained chromatin in interphase nuclei of buccal epithelium. We studied data on 130 patients: 68 patients with breast cancer, 33 patients with fibro adenomatosis and 29 healthy individuals containing in average data on 52 nuclei of buccal epithelium. The data set consists of 20256 images of interphase nuclei of buccal epithelium (6752 nuclei scanned without filter, through a yellow filter and through a violet filter). Each image consists of three channels: red, green, blue, as well as grey halftones. Fractal dimension was determined by the box-counting method. The classification was made by a novel method of segmentation, filtration and binarization of images and a novel measure of homogeneity of random samples. We call homogeneous samples that belong to the same population, i.e., following the same distribution. Results: the maximal accuracy of proposed screening test for breast cancer among several variants of nearest neighbors' methods and color channels more than 90%. Conclusion: novel

Applied Intelligence for Medical Image Analysis. Aarti, Raju Pal, Mukesh Saraswat, & Himanshu Mittal (Eds.)

method of breast cancer screening using fractal dimension of Feulgen-stained chromatin is very perspective and precise.

4.1 INTRODUCTION

In 2018, it was estimated that there were over 2 million new cases of breast cancer, which was more than 25% of all cancers in women.[1] Therefore, the task of noninvasive diagnosis of breast cancer is extremely important. Our approach to breast cancer screening is based on two phenomena: (1) malignancy-associated changes (MAC) in chromatin of interphase nuclei of buccal epithelium in women suffering from breast cancer, and (2) fractal packing of chromatin in a nucleus. MAC in nontumor cells were considered as diagnostic factors in papers of Susnik[2] and Us-Krasovec,[3] Ganina,[4,5] and Boroday.[6,7] These papers proved that MAC may be used for developing noninvasive methods for cancer detection.

In 2009, a team of authors[8] have discovered that DNA in a nucleus is packed as a 3D Peano curve. This fractal packing must be reflected in distribution of chromatin in the nucleus. Thus, we may suppose that the fractal dimension of chromatin in the buccal epithelium in healthy women and women with breast cancer, for example, fibroadenomatosis, is an informative diagnostic factor.

Now, the fractal dimension of chromatin is considered as a diagnostic and prognostic factor in endometrial cancer,[9] melanoma,[10] leukemia,[11,12] breast cancer,[13,14] and other diseases.[12–20] However, these papers considered only tumor cells.

Thus, the object of the chapter is a method of breast cancer screening using fractal analysis of Feulgen-stained chromatin in buccal epithelium. This chapter is organized as follows: Section 4.1 surveys papers on MAC in buccal epithelium. Section 4.2 represents the experimental methods and materials. Section 4.3 describes the methods of segmentation, binarization, and filtration of images used. Section 4.4 contains the description of the fractal analysis of images. In Section 4.5, we propose a test for homogeneity of random samples used for patient classification. Section 4.6 contains the results and discussion. The last section summarizes our investigation.

4.2 EXPERIMENTAL METHODS AND MATERIALS

We studied a control dataset of 29 healthy women, a test dataset consisting of 68 women with breast cancer, and a test dataset consisting of 33 women with fibroadenomatosis with histologically confirmed diagnosis. In summary, we have analyzed 20,256 images. We obtained scrapes from the spinous layer of buccal epithelium, dried them at room temperature, fixated in the Nikiforovs mixture, and carried out the Feulgen staining. Optical density of the Feulgen-stained chromatin was investigated using a microscope, a digital zoom camera, and a computer. As a result, we obtained digital images of the chromatin represented as square matrices 160 × 160 pixels.

4.3 SEGMENTATION, BINARIZATION, AND FILTRATION

4.3.1 SEGMENTATION OF NUCLEI

Before making fractal analysis, it is necessary to perform preprocessing and segmentation of images. The task of image segmentation consists of the following subtasks:

1) Noise reduction
2) Background separation
3) Isolation of a single-cell nucleus

The first and second subtasks are solved by means of traditional image filtering algorithms, and the second subtask is solved by means of the Otsu binarization algorithm. In the general case, if the image contains different objects (e.g., nuclei and artifacts), the third subtask is very difficult to solve by deterministic algorithms, because objects can overlap, touch each other, and have completely different shapes, colors, and dimensions. For example, Xie et al.[21] used neural networks to classify and segment cell images. We assume that the radii of these nuclei are approximately equal and we may use algorithms based on morphological operations, distance transformation, and watershed algorithm, which will be discussed in detail below.

4.3.1.1 NOISE REDUCTION AND MEDIAN FILTRATION

We reduced noise using a median filter.[22] Figure 4.1 shows how the noise level and image clarity change depending on the size of the filter window $k = 2r + 1$. It can be seen that at $k = 3$, the image is minimally devoid of noise, and the texture of the core is almost completely preserved. At $k = 13$, the contours of the cell nucleus stand out very well and the image is completely devoid of noise, but the texture of the nucleus is almost completely lost. Therefore, at different stages of the analysis, the median filters with different window sizes can be used. For example, when segmenting images, it is appropriate to use a large filter window, because at this stage, we are more interested in contours of objects, and when classifying (healthy, breast cancer, or fibroadenomatosis), it is better to use a small filter window as possible, because we are interested in the texture of the interphase nucleus of the buccal epithelial cell.

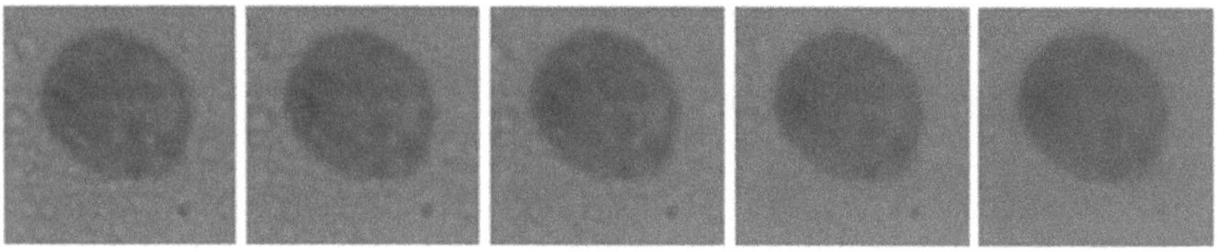

FIGURE 4.1 The images of Feulgen-stained chromatin (in a gray scale) after median filtration.

4.3.1.2 BACKGROUND SEGMENTATION AND BINARIZATION BY OTSU

The next step of image processing is to separate background from foreground objects. To achieve this goal, the algorithm of image binarization by Otsu is suitable.[23] Let the pixels of the image take values in 256 levels of gray color. Denote the number of pixels with value i as n_i and the general number of pixels as N. We must divide pixels into background and foreground pixels using some parameter k. As background ones, we will classify pixels with values $\{1, 2, \ldots, k\}$, and as foreground ones, we will classify pixels as the levels $\{k+1, k+2, \ldots, 256\}$. Let $h_b(k)$ and $h_f(k)$ be the relative frequencies of background and foreground pixels corresponding to the level k. Hence, $h_b(k) = \frac{1}{N}\sum_{i=0}^{k} n_i$, $h_f(k) = 1 - h_b$.

The Otsu method finds a threshold k that minimizes an intraclass variance, that is, a weighted sum of variances of two classes:

$$\sigma_\omega^2(k) = \sigma_b^2(k)h_b(k) + \sigma_f^2(k)h_f(k) \to \min,$$

where $\sigma_b^2(k)$ and $\sigma_f^2(k)$ are the variances of background and foreground brightness with respect to the threshold k. As Otsu has shown, the minimization of an intraclass variance is equivalent to the maximization of interclass variance:

$$\sigma_b^2(k) = h_b(k)h_f(k)(\mu_b(k) - \mu_f(k))^2 \to \max,$$

where $\mu_b(k)$ and $\mu_f(k)$ are the arithmetic mean of the background and foreground brightness with respect to the threshold k:

$$\mu_b(k) = \frac{1}{Nh_b(k)} \sum_{i=0}^{t-1} in_i, \quad \mu_f(k) = \frac{1}{Nh_f(k)} \sum_{i=0}^{256} in_i - \mu_b(k)\frac{h_b(k)}{h_f(k)}.$$

ALGORITHM 4.1 Binarization by Otsu.

Input: An $m \cdot n$ matrix (the initial image)

Output: Threshold k

Find a histogram n_i of the initial image and the relative frequency $N(i) = n_i/N$ of every level of the brightness of the initial image.

Compute the initial values $h_b(0)$, $h_f(0)$, $\mu_b(0)$ and $\mu_f(0)$.

Assign $\sigma_{\max}^2 \leftarrow 0$.

for $k = 1$ up to L do

Update $h_b(k)$, $h_f(k)$, $\mu_b(k)$ and $\mu_f(k)$.

Compute $\sigma_b^2(k) = h_b(k)h_f(k)(\mu_b(k) - \mu_f(k))^2$.

If $\sigma_b^2(k) \geq \sigma_{\max}^2(k)$, then

Assign $\sigma_{\max}^2 \leftarrow \sigma_b^2(k)$.

Assign $k \leftarrow \sigma_{\max}^2$.

The nonsmooth contours of the interphase nuclei of cells after binarization as well as inaccuracies in some regions of the image will be discussed in detail below.

4.3.1.3 BINARY MORPHOLOGICAL OPERATIONS ON IMAGE

In binary morphology,[24] a set of pixels is considered as a subset of $\mathbb{R}^d$ or $\mathbb{Z}^d(k)$. Morphology operations are applied to images together with a given structural element, or core, which determines the nature of the operation. The following structural element is most often used for image processing:

$$B = \{ (-1; -1); (-1; 0); (-1; 1); (0; -1); (0; 0); (0; 1);$$
$$(1; -1); (1; 0); (1; 1)\}:$$

There are two main morphological operations: erosion and dilation. The erosion operation is specified as $A \ominus B = \{z \in \mathbb{Z}^d \mid B_z \subseteq A\}$, where A is an image, B is a structural element, and B_z is the translation of the vector z, that is, $B_z = \{b + z \mid b \in B\}$ $\forall z \in \mathbb{Z}^d$. The idea is as follows. A structural element slides through an image. A point of a binary image has value 1 only if all points of a structural element have value 1; otherwise, it is equal to 0. Due to this operation, we reduced a foreground object, removed small noises, and separated two overlapped objects.

The dilation is specified as $A \oplus B = \bigcup_{b \in B} A_b$. This operation is the opposite of erosion. Here, a pixel of a binary image is equal to 1 if at least one pixel in the core is equal to 1. Thus, the white increases the image area or the size of the foreground object increases. Typically, when you need to remove noise around an object, you first use a narrowing operation and then the dilation. Dilation is necessary because erosion, in addition to removing white noise, reduces our object. Other operations are specified using the basic operations of erosion and dilation. For example, the operation of morphological opening is $A \circ B = (A \ominus B) \oplus B$ or $A \circ B = \bigcup_{B_z \subseteq A} B_z$.

4.3.1.4 DISTANCE TRANSFORMATION

Distance transformation is an operation of mathematical morphology that maps each foreground pixel of the binary image $E \subseteq \mathbb{Z}^d$ to the distance of this point from the nearest background pixel (which does not belong to E). The Manhattan distance is a distance that is most often used for binary images:

$$DT(z) = \inf_{(x,y)} \left(|x - z_x| + |y - z_y| \right),$$

where $z = (z_x, z_y) \in E \subseteq F \subseteq \mathbb{Z}^d$.

In our case, the result of this operation can be interpreted as the probability that the pixel z belongs to the interphase nucleus of a buccal epithelial cell. Thus, we can specify an empirical rule according to which we will take certain pixels as exactly belonging to the cell nucleus:

$$DT(z) \geq \alpha \sup_{s \in E} DT(s) \Rightarrow z \text{ is exactly belonging to the cell nucleus.}$$

Denote the set that satisfies this inequality as $\wedge$. The multiplier $\langle = 0.475$ was chosen experimentally based on the studied data. The assumption is also used here that all cell nuclei have approximately the same size, and therefore, the centers of these cells will be at approximately the same distance from the background points. If the data are collected under different conditions, it is necessary to choose another multiplier.

In $\wedge$ the nuclei do not touch, thanks to the selected parameter $\langle$, that is, segmentation correctly handles situations when cells touch or partially overlap. Let us call an image obtained as a result of an dilation of a binary image as *D*, and a result of an opening of a binary image as *O*. Obviously, that all the pixels that equal to zero in $\wedge$ are the background pixels. Thus, we must look for nuclei only among the points of *O*, which equal to zero.

Using the recursive algorithm proposed in Ref. [25], we can compute the distance transformation in two iterations. For complete detection of individual cells, we use the watershed algorithm.

4.3.1.5 WATERSHED ALGORITHM

The watershed algorithm considers a single-channel image as a topographic map, where the pixel value reflects the height of this point. Starting from the points of local minima (or from the given points), each basin is filled with liquids of different colors. The liquid level rises, thus there comes a moment when two liquids of different colors begin to mix. To avoid this, borders are being built between the basins. Boundaries are constructed until the liquid level is higher than the highest point of the map. The constructed boundaries are the results of segmentation.

We use this idea to segment cell nuclei. We will paint each connected component of Ω in a certain color. Let us call such segmentation a set of markers. Let's denote $\wedge = E \setminus D$.

We will also paint the connected set $\wedge$ consisting of the background pixels in a certain color. The following set remains unpainted:

$$N = D \setminus \wedge.$$

ALGORITHM 4.2 Mayer watershed algorithm with given markers.

Input: An $m \cdot n$ matrix and a set of markers

Output: A segmented image

0. We will consider that flooding begins with pixels of markers.
1. Neighboring pixels of each marker are added to the priority queue, where the priority level depends on a gradient.
2. Consider a pixel with the lowest brightness. If neighboring pixels are already colored and have the same color, then we color this pixel in the color of the neighbors. Otherwise, neighbors are added to the queue.
3. Repeat step 2 until the queue is empty.
4. Uncolored pixels form watershed boundaries.

4.3.1.6 FINAL SEGMENTATION ALGORITHM

Consider the final algorithm for segmentation.

ALGORITHM 4.3: Nucleus segmentation.

Input: An matrix $m \cdot n$ (an image)

Output: A colored image with highlighted cells

1. Transform the image to the gray scale
2. Carry out the median filtration of gray-scaled image with window size $r = 2$.
3. Carry out Otsu binarization.
4. Carry out the morphological opening with kernel $9 \cdot 9$ in two iterations (the set O).
5. Carry out the morphological dilation with kernel $9 \cdot 9$ in two iterations (the set D).
6. Compute the distance transformation for the set O.
7. $\wedge \leftarrow z$ minimizing the Manhattan distance.
8. $U = D \setminus \wedge$.
9. Mark connected components of $\wedge$ and E / Ω.
10. Execute the watershed algorithm.
11. Normalize an image.

In some cases, it is important to make sure that the input data are normalized. In our case, images can be formed in slightly different conditions. This may affect the recognition accuracy. Assign the background normalization of the histogram for the image of one cell nucleus to the background of the image so that the pixels of the nucleus take values from

0 to 255. Using the previous results, we will remove the background from the image. The cell nucleus is normalized by histogram equalization.

4.3.2 FILTRATION OF IMAGES

According to Lyashko et al.,[27] the image filtering based on the Petunin ellipsoids has many advantages over the median filtering. In the case of image filtering of interphase cell nuclei, this method better preserves the shape of the texture. Therefore, it can be used to preprocess data for fractal analysis.

4.3.2.1 PETUNIN ELLIPSOIDS

Suppose we have a set of points $M = \{x_1, x_2, \ldots, x_n\}$, where $x_i \in \mathbb{R}^m$. Find the points x_l and x_k such that

$$\sup_{x_i, x_j \in M} \|x_i - x_j\| = \|x_l - x_k\|.$$

In other words, the segment $L = [x_1, x_k]$ is a diameter of M. Rotate and transfer coordinate axes so that the diameter L be aligned along the axis $O_{x_1'}$, where $x_1', x_2', \ldots, x_n'$ are the coordinates of the set M in the new coordinate system.

We construct the smallest rectangular parallelepiped in $\mathbb{R}^m$, which would contain elements of the set $M' = \{x_1', x_2', \ldots, x_n'\}$. Compressing this smallest rectangular parallelepiped, we map its points in a hypercube. Find the center x_0 of the hypercube and calculate the distances $r_1, r_2, \ldots, r_n$ from it to every point. Then, find maximal $r_1, r_2, \ldots, r_n$ and construct hyperballs with a center x_0 and radii r_i. Executing back stretching, rotating, and translation, we obtain a concentric system of Petunins ellipsoids for the set M. Outer ellipsoid is called the Petunin ellipsoid covering given set of points. For a system of concentric ellipsoids, the properties are the consequences of Hills work[28] and are described and proved in detail in Lyashko et al.[29]

4.3.2.2 IMAGE FILTERING BASED ON PETUNIN ELLIPSOIDS

Suppose we have an image at the input, each pixel of which has d channels. The image is considered a mapping that maps every coordinate to a d-channel value. For each pixel of the image, we consider a few more pixels, the coordinates of which are in the radius r from this pixel. We construct a family of concentric Petunin ellipsoids for the set of values of these pixels, and in the output image, we assign to the pixel with the same coordinates a value that corresponds to the inner (or central) ellipsoid. The detailed algorithm is as follows.

ALGORITHM 4.4 Filtering by Petunin.

Input: An $m \cdot n$ matrix, size of filter window r

Output: A filtered image

for $i = 1$ up to m do

  for $j = 1$ up to n do

    $D \leftarrow$ an infinite segment;

      for $k = -r$ up to r do

        for $l = -r$ up to r do

          for $q = -r$ up to r do

            for $p = -r$ up to r do

              If $\|D\| < \|X_{i+k; j+1} - X_{i+q; j+p}\|$ then $D \leftarrow [X_{i+k; j+1}; X_{i+q; j+p}]$

Construct a family of concentrated Petunin ellipsoids of diameter D.

$Y_{i;j} \leftarrow$ the value corresponding to the inner ellipsoid.

4.3.2.3 FAST ALGORITHM BASED ON DYNAMIC PROGRAMMING

Despite the advantages of the filtering based on the Petunin ellipsoids over the median filtering, it has a serious drawback. The time complexity of the algorithm is $O(mnr^4)$. For comparison, the asymptotic time complexity of the fast median filtration algorithm or the Gaussian filter is $O(\min\{m, n\} r^2 + mnr)$. Thus, for large kernel sizes (e.g., $r > 10$) and a large volume of images, the image filtering based on Petunin ellipsoids works much more slowly than other filtration algorithms. The main reason is the slow search for diameter. There are many fast algorithms for finding the furthest points in a set in a multidimensional space. For example, Har-Peled proposed a heuristic algorithm for finding the diameter.[30] In Malandain and Boissonnat,[31] Malandain and Boissonnat proposed a deterministic algorithm that allows us to find the diameter for time $O(n\log n)$, where n is the number of points of the set. The disadvantage of these algorithms when used for a filter based on Petunin ellipsoids is that, despite the smaller asymptotics, these algorithms work at a small number of points no faster than a naive algorithm (exhaustive search).

We noticed that when we move the filter window, we repeat some calculations. If we can perform calculations more optimally (without repetitions), then we will be able to filter the image faster. Thus, we offer an algorithm based on dynamic programming, which significantly speeds up the diameter search process.

Let us introduce a data structure, which we will call the "two-dimensional queue that store the diameter." This structure is a tuple $(H; p)$, where p is the coordinate of the center of the filter window relative to the image X, and H is a table of size $(2r + 1) \cdot (2r + 1)$, each element of which stores the diameter of the set of points corresponding pixels that fall into the filter below or to the right, ік:

$$H_{i,j} = \|D(X_{y,x}|x\in[(p_x + i), (p_x + r)]_Z; y\in[(p_y + j); (p_y + r)]_Z\})\|, i; j = -r\ldots r$$

where D is the diameter of the set and $X_{y,x}$ is the d-dimensional value of the pixel with coordinates (y,x).

It is obvious that $H_{-r,-r}$ stores the diameter of the set of points of pixel values that fall into the filter window. We describe the algorithm for updating table H when moving the filter to the right. The algorithm is set in a similar way when moving the filter down.

ALGORITHM 4.5 Updating table H when moving the filter window to the right.

Input: Image X, kernel radius (size of filter window) r, two-dimensional queue that stores the diameter $(H;p)$ corresponding to the window

Output: Two-dimensional queue storing the diameter $(H_0; p_0)$ corresponding to the window after shifting to the right by 1 pixel

$$H'_{r,r} \leftarrow 0$$

for $i = r-1$ down to $-r$ do

$$H'_{r,r} \leftarrow \max\left\{\max\left\{\left\|X_{p_y+i,p_x+r} - X_{p_y+j,p_x+r}\right\| \ \forall k \in i\ldots r\right\}, H'_{i+1,r}\right\}$$

for $i = r-1$ down to $-r$ do

$$H'_{r,r} \leftarrow \max\left\{\max\left\{\left\|X_{p_y+i,p_x+r} - X_{p_y+j,p_x+r}\right\| \ \forall k \in i\ldots r\right\}, H'_{i+1,j}, H'_{i,j+1}\right\}.$$

Let us also describe an algorithm for calculating $(H; p)$, knowing $(H^{left}; p^{left})$ and $(H^{top}; p^{top})$, where $p^{left} = (p_y; p_x - 1)$ and $p^{top} = (p_y - 1; p_x)$, that is, knowing the queues that correspond to the windows one pixel above or to the left.

ALGORITHM 4.6 Calculation of table H knowing the corresponding tables on the left and above.

Input: Image X, kernel radius (size of filter window) r, two-dimensional queues storing the diameter $(H^{left}; p^{left})$ and $(H^{top}; p^{top})$ corresponding to the window to the left and above, respectively

Output: Two-dimensional queue that stores the diameter $(H; p)$

$$H_{r,r} \leftarrow 0$$

for $i = r$ down to $-r$ do

for $j = r$ down to $-r$ do

$$H_{ij} = \max\left\{H^{left}_{i,j+1}, H^{top}_{i+1,j}, H_{i,j+1}, H_{i+1,j}, \left\|X_{p_y+r,p_x+r} - X_{p_y+i,p_x+j}\right\|\right\}.$$

It should be noted that in Algorithms 4.5 and 4.6 after each step of assigning the diameter value, the points of the ends of the diameter should also be saved in the table $D_{i,j}$. Below we describe the final algorithm for fast image filtering based on the family of concentric Petunin ellipsoids:

ALGORITHM 4.7 Fast filtration algorithm by Petunin.

Input: An $w \cdot h$ matrix, size of filter window r

Output: A filtered image Y

Calculate $(H_0; p_0 = (1; 1))$ as well as the corresponding segment L_0;

for $i = 1$ up to h do

By Algorithm 4.5, calculate $(H^{i,1}, p^{i,1} = (i; 1))$ and the corresponding segment $L^{i,1}$.

Construct a system of concentric Petunin ellipsoids of the diameter $L^{i,1}$.

$Y_{i,1} \leftarrow$ the value corresponding to the inner (or central) ellipsoid;

for $j = 1$ up to w do

By Algorithm 4.5, calculate $(H^{1,j}; p^{1,j} = (1,j))$ and the corresponding segment $L^{1,j}$.

Construct a family of concentric Petunin ellipsoids of the diameter $L^{1,j}$.

$Y_{1,j} \leftarrow$ the value corresponding to the inner ellipsoid.

for $i = 1$ up to h do

for $j = 1$ up to w do

By Algorithm 4.6 calculate $(H^{i,j}; p^{i,j})$ and the corresponding segment $L^{i,j}$.

Construct a system of concentric Petunin ellipsoids of the diameter $L^{i,j}$.

$Y_{i,j} \leftarrow$ the value corresponding to the inner (or central) ellipsoid.

It is obvious that Algorithm 4.5 has the asymptotic time complexity $O(r^3)$, and Algorithm 4.6 has the asymptotic time complexity $O(r^2)$. Then, the asymptotic time complexity of Algorithm 4.7 is equal to $O(r^4 + r^3 (w + h) + whr^2)$. Since r is much smaller than the size of the image $w \cdot h$, the asymptotic time complexity of Algorithm 4.7 can be estimated as $O(whr^2)$, that is, it is equal to the asymptotic time complexity of the usual median filtration algorithm.

4.4 FRACTAL ANALYSIS OF CHROMATIN

Next, we calculate the fractal dimension of preprocessed images.

4.4.1 *THEORETICAL BASIS*

To describe the concept of a fractal, we must first define the Hausdorff dimension.[32] Consider a bounded set in a metric space X. Let $\sum > 0$. We shall call a not more than the countable family $\{\omega_i\}_{i \in I}$ of subsets of X as an $\sum$-coverage of the set $\wedge$ if

1) $\Omega \subset \bigcup_{i \in I} \omega_i$,

2) $\forall i \in I : |\omega_i| < \varepsilon$,

where $|\omega_i| < \varepsilon$ is the diameter of ω_i.

Let $\langle > 0$ and $\Theta = \{\omega_i\}_{i \in I}$ be a coverage of $\wedge$. The size of the covering is $F_\alpha(\theta) \triangleq \sum_{i \in I} |\omega_i|^\alpha$. Denote by $M_\alpha^\varepsilon(\Omega)$ the minimal size of an $\sum$-coverage of $\wedge$, such that $M_\alpha^\varepsilon(\Omega) \triangleq \inf(F_\alpha(\theta))$, where the infimum is taken on all $\sum$-coverings of $\wedge$. As $\sum$ is decreasing, $M_\alpha^\varepsilon(\Omega)$ does not decrease since a set of possible $\sum$-coverages is decreasing also. So, there exists a limit $M_\alpha(\Omega) = \lim_{\varepsilon \to 0+} M_\alpha^\varepsilon(\Omega)$.

The quantity $M_{\langle}(\wedge)$ is called the Hausdorff $\langle$-measure of the set. Also, any set $\wedge$ has a threshold $\langle_0$ satisfying the following conditions:

1. $M_{\langle}(\wedge) = 0$ for all $\langle > \langle_0$.
2. $M_{\langle}(\wedge) = +\infty$ for all $\langle < \langle_0$.

The value of M_0 () can be zero, infinitely positive, or infinite. The number $\langle_0$ is a Hausdorf dimension of the set $\wedge$ and following Mandelbrot,[32] we shall say that a set is fractal if its Hausdorff dimension is larger than its topological dimension.

4.4.2 BOX-COUNTING ALGORITHM

Self-similarity of images is described by fractal dimension.[33] The Hausdorff dimension is rather a theoretical concept but the box-counting method is usually used in practice.[34] This method consists in calculating some function $M_{™}(\wedge)$ for an arbitrary positive ™. If $M_{™}(\wedge) \propto$ ™-D, the fractal dimension $\wedge$ is D. Thus, the box-counting dimension of $\wedge$ is $\dim_B \Omega = D = \lim_{\delta \to 0} \frac{\log(M_\delta(\Omega))}{-\log(\delta)}$, where $M_{™}(\wedge)$ is the number of hypercubes with sides ™ covering $\wedge$.

As noted in the previous section, the use of the box-counting algorithm requires verification of the ratio $M_{™}(\wedge) \propto$ ™-D, and hence the calculation of the linear regression. The angular coefficient of this line is equal to $\dim_B$. We will look for a linear regression by the method of the best root-mean-squared approximation (Figure 4.2).

4.5 METHODS OF PATIENTS CLASSIFICATION

To test the hypothesis that fractal dimensions of cancer and healthy patients have different distributions, we used the p-statistics (see Klyushin and Petunin[35]). It uses the Hills assumption $A_{(n)}$[28] about independent identically distributed exchangeable random values $x_1, x_2, \ldots, x_n$ drawn from a distribution without ties. This assumption states that $P\left(x \in \left(x_{(i)}, x_{(j)}\right)\right) = \frac{j-i}{n+1}$, where $j > i$ and $x_{(i)}$ is the ith order statistics. Let $x_1, x_2, \ldots, x_n$ and $y_1, y_2, \ldots, y_n$ are drawn from the same distribution. Denote as $A_{ij}^{(k)}$ an event $\left\{x_{(i)} < y_k < x_{(j)}\right\}$. If $j > i$, then $P\left(A_{ij}^{(k)}\right) = \frac{j-i}{n+1}$.

The lower and upper limits of the Wilson interval $I_{ij}^{(n)}$ for an unknown probability of the event $A_{ij}^{(k)}$ are $p_{ij}^{(1)} = \frac{h_{ij}n + g^2/2 - g\sqrt{h_{ij}(1-h_{ij})n + g^2/4}}{n+g^2}$, $p_{ij}^{(2)} = \frac{h_{ij}n + g^2/2 - g\sqrt{h_{ij}(1-h_{ij})n + g^2/4}}{n+g^2}$, where h_{ij} is the relative frequency of $A_{ij}^{(k)}$. If $g = 3$, then the confidence level of $I_{ij}^{(n)}$ is greater than 0.95.[35] The p-statistics is the relative frequency of the event $\left\{\frac{j-i}{n+1} \in I_{ij}^{(n)}\right\}$.

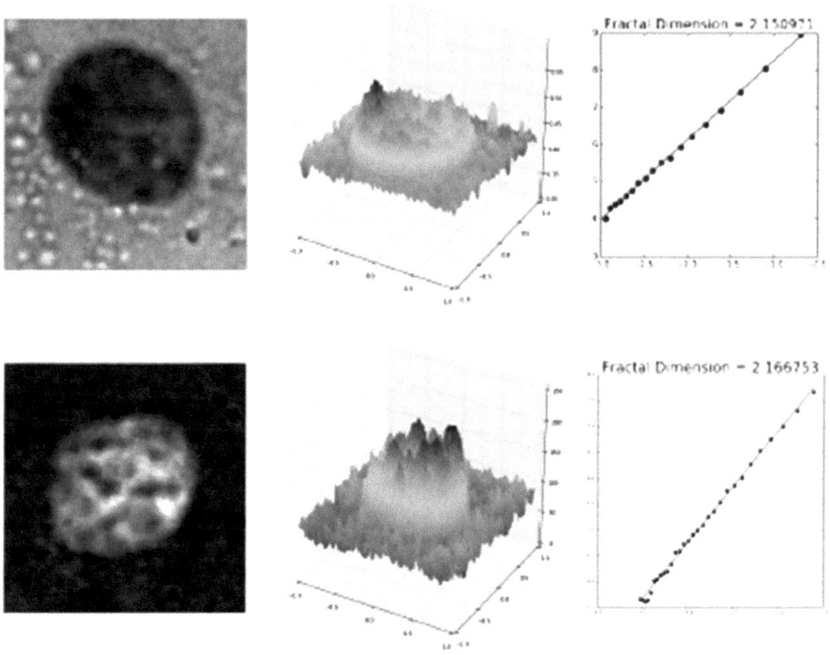

FIGURE 4.2 Estimation of fractal dimension using the box-counting method.

Using the method of k-nearest neighbors to classify patients, we used the compactness hypothesis stated by Braverman[36]: the vast majority of objects of the same class are closer to each other than to objects of concurrent class and lie in a domain with a relatively simple boundary. The essence of this method for the classification of the element x is that from the training sample, we choose k elements closest to x in the sense of p-statistics and refer x to the dominant class of these k elements.

4.6 RESULTS AND DISCUSSION

Tables 4.1–4.6 demonstrate the results of the diagnostics between the control and the joined sample of breast cancer and fibroadenomatosis patients using cross-validation. Let us introduce a parameter $S = M/N$, where M is the number of training samples and N is the number of samples in the dataset.

TABLE 4.1 Dependence of the Average Sensitivity (after Cross-Validation) on *S* and the Number of Neighbors for the Red Channel.

S	Numbers of neighbors					
	6	**7**	**8**	**9**	**10**	**12**
0.5	87.43	81.42	88.86	83.71	87.42	85.43
0.6	83.93	83.93	86.78	83.93	87.14	84.29
0.7	85.23	88.10	89.05	90.00	87.62	90.00
0.8	87.14	84.29	90.00	89.29	86.43	93.57
0.9	82.86	82.86	85.71	84.29	91.42	84.26

TABLE 4.2 Dependence of the Average Specificity (after Cross-Validation) on *S* and the Number of Neighbors for the Red Channel.

S	Numbers of neighbors					
	6	**7**	**8**	**9**	**10**	**12**
0.5	64.00	74.00	63.33	74.67	62.00	63.33
0.6	65.83	70.83	65.33	69.17	64.17	68.33
0.7	68.89	72.22	58.89	71.11	73.33	68.89
0.8	71.67	65.00	68.33	66.67	73.33	70.00
0.9	83.33	83.33	53.33	73.33	66.67	66.67

TABLE 4.3 Dependence of the Average Sensitivity (after Cross-Validation) on *S* and the Number of Neighbors for the Green Channel.

S	Numbers of neighbors					
	6	**7**	**8**	**9**	**10**	**12**
0.5	90.86	85.14	89.71	86.86	88.29	87.71
0.6	87.50	83.57	91.07	83.57	90.36	88.93
0.7	81.90	85.71	90.95	87.62	89.04	83.81
0.8	81.43	83.57	88.57	80.00	89.29	91.43
0.9	84.29	87.14	88.57	87.14	85.71	82.86

TABLE 4.4 Dependence of the Average Specificity (after Cross-Validation) on *S* and the Number of Neighbors for the Green Channel.

S	Numbers of neighbors					
	6	7	8	9	10	12
0.5	63.33	71.33	67.33	67.33	66.67	60.67
0.6	61.67	69.17	71.67	70.00	67.50	65.00
0.7	71.11	70.00	61.11	77.78	66.67	70.00
0.8	71.67	75.00	70.00	76.67	63.33	71.67
0.9	60.00	63.33	70.00	76.67	73.33	70.00

TABLE 4.5 Dependence of the Average Sensitivity (after Cross-Validation) on *S* and the Number of Neighbors for the Blue Channel.

S	Numbers of neighbors					
	6	7	8	9	10	12
0.5	88.86	80.29	86.86	85.71	89.71	86.57
0.6	84.29	84.64	87.14	86.43	90.36	86.43
0.7	88.57	85.71	91.90	80.95	90.00	89.53
0.8	84.29	80.71	89.29	83.57	90.71	89.29
0.9	82.86	81.43	91.43	77.14	92.80	81.43

TABLE 4.6 Dependence of the Average Specificity (after Cross-Validation) on *S* and the Number of Neighbors for the Blue Channel.

S	Numbers of neighbors					
	6	7	8	9	10	12
0.5	62.67	74.67	66.67	69.33	61.33	62.00
0.6	66.67	73.33	65.00	69.17	64.17	67.50
0.7	60.00	68.89	62.22	71.11	61.11	60.00
0.8	55.00	76.67	65.00	66.67	61.67	68.33
0.9	76.67	86.67	70.00	73.33	70.00	53.33

We see several facts: (1) the best average sensitivity (93.57) is achieved for the red channel when $S = 0.8$ and the number of the neighbors is 12 (see Table 3.1); (2) the best average specificity (83.33) is achieved for the red channel when $S = 0.9$ and the number of the neighbors is 6 (see Table 1.1); (3) varying of S has very weak effect on the sensitivity and specificity;

and (4) varying of the numbers of neighbors has very weak effect on the sensitivity and specificity.

These observations may be explained by statistical homogeneity of the dataset. If the samples from the dataset are homogeneous, then the p-statistics does not vary in the wide range and increasing of the parameter S and the number of the neighbors weakly effect on the results of diagnostics. Meantime, the accuracy of this method is rather high and has excellent clinic perspectives when used properly.

4.7 CONCLUSION

New method of breast cancer screening using box-counting dimension of nuclear chromatin in buccal epithelium stained by Feulgen has high sensitivity, specificity, and accuracy. The fractal dimension is an informative diagnostic index that allows detecting breast cancer with high precision. The new methods of segmentation and filtrations proposed in the chapter are useful tools for preprocessing images that improve the accuracy of diagnosis. The method of breast cancer screening proposed in the chapter is noninvasive, easy for implementation, and precise; thus, it could be recommended as a perspective tool for breast cancer screening. The future study will be aimed on the differential diagnosis between the breast cancer and fibroadenomatosis that still is an open problem.

KEYWORDS

- **malignancy-associated changes**
- **buccal epithelium**
- **segmentation**
- **filtration**
- **binarization**
- **breast cancer**
- **image analysis**
- **fractal dimension**

REFERENCES

1. Bray, F.; Ferlay, J.; Soerjomataram, I.; Siegel, R. L.; Torre, L. A.; Jemal, A. Global Cancer Statistics 2018: GLOBOCAN Estimates of Incidence and Mortality Worldwide for 36 Cancers in 185 Countries. *CA Cancer J Clin.* **2018,** *68* (6), 394–424. DOI: 10.3322/caac.21492.
2. Susnik, B.; Worth; A., LeRiche; J.; Palcic, B. Malignancy-Associated Changes in the Breast: Changes in Chromatin Distribution in Epithelial Cells in Normal-Appearing Tissue Adjacent to Carcinoma. *Anal. Quant. Cytol. Histol.* **1995,** *17* (1), 62–68.
3. Us-Krasovec, M.; Erzen, J.; Zganec, M.; et al. Malignancy Associated Changes In Epithelial Cells of Buccal Mucosa: A Potential Cancer Detection Test. *Anal. Quant. Cytol. Histol.* **2005,** *27* (5), 254–262.
4. Ganina, K. P.; Boroday, N. V.; Petunin, Y. I. Klyushin DA Quantitative Evaluation of Malignancy-Associated Changes of DNA in the Nuclei of Buccal Epithelium in Fibroadenoma, Fibroadenomatosis and Breast Cancer. *Exp. Oncol.* **1998,** *20* (2), 130–134.
5. Klyushin, D. A.; Petunin, Y. I.; Andrushkiw, R. I., Boroday, N. V.; Ganina, K. P. Analysis of Malignancy-Associated DNA Changes in the Nuclei of Buccal Epithelium in the Pathology of the Thyroid and Mammary Glands. *Ann. N. Y. Acad. Sci.* **2002,** *980* (1), 1–12. DOI: 10.1111/j.1749-6632.2002.tb04884.x.
6. Andrushkiw, R. I.; Boroday, N. V.; Klyushin, D. A.; Petunin, Yu, I. *Computer-Aided Cytogenetic Method of Cancer Diagnosis*; Nova Publishers: New York, 2007.
7. Boroday, N.; Chekhun, V.; Golubeva, E.; Klyushin, D. In Vitro and In Vivo Densitometric Analysis of DNA Content and Chromatin Texture in Nuclei of Tumor Cells under the Influence of a Nanocomposite and Magnetic Field. *Adv. Cancer Res. Treat.* **2016**. Article ID 706183. DOI: 10.5171/2016.706183.
8. Lieberman-Aiden, E.; et al. Comprehensive Mapping of Long-Range Interactions Reveals Folding Principles of the Human Genome. *Science* **2009,** *326* (5959), 289–293. DOI: 10.1126/science.1181369.
9. Bikou, O.; et al. Fractal Dimension as a Diagnostic Tool of Complex Endometrial Hyperplasia and Well-Differentiated Endometrioid Carcinoma. *In Vivo* **2016,** *30* (5), 681–690.
10. Bedin, V.; et al. Fractal Dimension of Chromatin is an Independent Prognostic Factor for Survival in Melanoma. *BMC Cancer* **2010,** *10*, 260, doi: 10.1186/1471-2407-10-260
11. Adam, R.; Silva, R.; Pereira, F.; et al. The Fractal Dimension of Nuclear Chromatin as a Prognostic Factor in Acute Precursor B Lymphoblastic Leukemia. *Cell Oncol* **2006,** *28*, 55–59. DOI: 10.1155/2006/409593.
12. Mashiah, A.; Wolach, O.; Sandbank, J.; et al. Lymphoma and Leukemia Cells Possess Fractal Dimensions That Correlate with Their Interpretation in Terms of Fractal Biological Features. *Acta Haematol.* **2008,** *119*, 142–150. DOI: 10.1159/000125551.
13. Einstein, A.; Wu, H.; Sanchez, M.; Gil, J. Fractal Characterization of Chromatin Appearance for Diagnosis in Breast Cytology. *J. Pathol.* **1998,** *185*, 366–381. DOI: 10.1002/(SICI)1096-9896(199808)185:4<366::AID-PATH122>3.0.CO;2-C.
14. Losa, G.; Castelli, C. Nuclear Patterns of Human Breast Cancer Cells During Apoptosis: Characterization by Fractal Dimension and (GLCM) Co-occurrence Matrix Statistics. *Cell Tissue Res.* **2005,** *322*, 257–267. DOI: 10.1007/s00441-005-0030-2.

15. Losa, G. Fractals and Their Contribution to Biology and Medicine. *Medicographia* **2012,** *34*, 365–374.
16. Metze, K. Fractal Dimension of Chromatin and Cancer Prognosis. *Epigenomics* **2010,** *2* (5), 601–604. DOI: 10.1080/14737159.2019.1597707.
17. Metze, K.; Adam, R., Florindo, J. B. The Fractal Dimension of Chromatin ↓ a Potential Molecular Marker for Carcinogenesis, Tumor Progression and Prognosis. *Expert Rev. Mol. Diagn.* **2019,** *19* (4), 299–312. DOI: 10.1080/14737159.2019.1597707.
18. Nikolaou, N., Papamarkos, N. Color Image Retrieval Using a Fractal Signature Extraction Technique. *Eng. Appl. Artif. Intell.* **2002,** *15* (1), 81–96. DOI: 10.1016/S0952-1976(02)00028-3.
19. Ohri, S.; Dey, P.; Nijhawan, R. Fractal Dimension in Aspiration Cytology Smears of Breast and Cervical Lesions. *Anal. Quant. Cytol. Histol.* **2004,** *26*:109–112.
20. Muniandy, S.; Stanlas, J. Modelling of Chromatin Morphologies in Breast Cancer Cells Undergoing Apoptosis Using Generalized Cauchy Field. *Comput. Med. Imaging Graph.* **2008,** *32*, 631–637. DOI: 10.1016/j.compmedimag.2008.07.003.
21. Xie, W.; Noble, J.; Zisserman, A. Microscopy Cell Counting and Detection with Fully Convolutional Regression Networks. *Comput. Methods Biomech. Biomed. Eng. Imaging Vis.* **2016,** *6* (3), 283–292. DOI: 10.1080/21681163.2016.1149104.
22. Perreault, S.; Hebert, P. Median Filtering in Constant Time. *IEEE Trans. Image Process.* **2007,** *16* (9) 2389–2394. DOI: 10.1109/TIP.2007.902329.
23. Otsu, N. A Threshold Selection Method from Gray-Level Histograms. *IEEE Trans. Syst. Man. Cybern. Syst.* **1979,** *9* (1), 62–66. DOI: 10.1109/TSMC.1979.4310076.
24. Serra, J. *Image Analysis and Mathematical Morphology*; Academic Press Inc.: Cambridge, MA, 1983.
25. Rosenfeld, A.; Pfaltz, J. Distance Functions in Digital Pictures. *Pattern Recogn.* **1968,** *1*, 33–61, DOI: 10.1016/0031-3203(68)90013-7.
26. Barnes, R.; Lehman, C.; Mulla, D. Priority-Flood: An Optimal Depression-Filling and Watershed-Labeling Algorithm for Digital Elevation Models. *Comput. Geosci.* **2014,** *62*, 117–127. DOI: 10.1016/j.cageo.2013.04.024.
27. Lyashko, S. I.; Klyushin, D. A.; Semenov, V. V.; Prysiazhna, M. V.; Shlykov, M. P. Nonparametric Ellipsoidal Approximation of Compact Sets of Random Points. In *Optimization and Its Applications in Control and Data Sciences. Springer Optimization and Its Applications*; Goldengorin, B., Ed.; Springer: Cham, 2016, Vol. 115. DOI: 10.1007/978-3-319-42056-1_11.
28. Hill, B. M. Posterior Distribution of Percentiles: Bayes' Theorem for Sampling from a Population. *J. Am. Stat. Assoc.* **1968,** *63* (322), 677–691. DOI: 10.1080/01621459.1968.11009286.
29. Lyashko, S. I., Klyushin, D. A.; Alexeyenko, V. V. Multivariate Ranking Using Elliptical Peeling. *Cybern. Syst. Anal.* **2013,** *49* (4), 511–516. DOI: 10.1007/s10559-013-9536-x.
30. Har-Peled S. A Practical Approach for Computing the Diameter of a Point Set. In *SCG '01: Proceedings of the 17th Annual Symposium on Computational Geometry*, 2001; pp 177–186. DOI: 10.1145/378583.378662.
31. Malandain, G.; Boissonnat, J.-D. Computing the Diameter of a Point Set. *Int. J. Comput. Geom. Appl.* **2002,** *12* (6), 498–509. DOI: 10.1142/S0218195902001006.
32. Mandelbrot, B. *The Fractal Geometry of Nature*; W. H. Freeman and Co.: New York, NY, 1982.

33. Voss, R. F. Random Fractal Forgeries. In *Fundamental Algorithms for Computer Graphics. NATO ASI Series (Series F: Computer and Systems Sciences)*; Earnshaw, R. A., Ed.; 1985; Springer: Berlin-Heidelberg; Vol 17, pp 805-835. DOI: 10.1007/978-3-642-84574-1_34.
34. Peleg, S.; Naor, J.; Hartley, R.; Avnir, D. Multiple Resolution Texture Analysis and Classification. *IEEE Trans Pattern Anal Mach Intell* **1984,** PAMI-6 (4), 518–523. DOI: 10.1109/TPAMI.1984.4767557.
35. Klyushin, D. A; Petunin, Y. I. A Nonparametric Test for the Equivalence of Populations Based on a Measure of Proximity of Samples. *Ukrainian Math. J.* **2003,** *55* (2), 181–198. DOI: 10.1023/A:1025495727612.
36. Arkadev, A. G.; Braverman, E. M. *Computers and Pattern Recognition*; Thompson Book Company: Stamford, CT, 1967.

CHAPTER 5

Polycystic Ovary Syndrome Classification Based on Machine Learning Techniques: A Comparative Analysis

NANCY GIRDHAR, PRIYA SINGH, and TISHA SINGHAL

Department of Computer Science and Technology, Amity University, Noida, India

ABSTRACT

Polycystic ovary syndrome (PCOS) is an ailment predominantly occurring in females of reproductive age ranging from 15 years to 45 years, that is, the time span between menopause and menarche. The root cause is unknown but medical symptoms show that the disease causes the excessive production of male hormone in the female body resulting in cysts in the ovaries of women. The disturbances in the hormones lead to various drastic symptoms including hirsutism, male pattern baldness, type 2 diabetes, endometrial cancer, and irregular menstrual cycle causing infertility and complications in pregnancy. This chapter focuses on the diagnosis classification of the syndrome on the selected set of features that are most associated with the disease adopting various machine learning algorithms. Algorithms applied to the dataset are logistic regression, Gaussian-naïve Bayes, *K*-nearest neighbors, random forest, decision tree classifier, and Xtreme gradient boosting and then a comparison is drawn of these machine learning algorithms to find out the best performing model in the classification of the PCOS patients.

Applied Intelligence for Medical Image Analysis. Aarti, Raju Pal, Mukesh Saraswat, & Himanshu Mittal (Eds.)

5.1 INTRODUCTION

Polycystic ovary syndrome (PCOS) is a condition which occurs due to the high secretion of male hormones in the body than normal. Poly means many and cysts are the immature follicles.[1] Nowadays, PCOS is a very common disorder of hormones among women; in every five women, one is suffering from PCOS. This syndrome affects the women lying between 15 and 44 years of age, that is, the lifespan between menarche and menopause.[2] Women that are suffering from PCOS have high chances to suffer from many other diseases such as diabetes, infertility, heart diseases, and obesity. So, it is very important to start the medication of PCOS at early stages to decrease these long-lasting side effect of the problem. There are many symptoms of PCOS, in which some common symptoms that every woman with PCOS suffers are acne, hirsutism, irregular menstrual cycle, and weight gain.[3] The exact cause of the problem has not been known till date. Some of the causes that are used by doctors to predict this problem are due to excess production of insulin, changes in hormones, and due to bad lifestyle. It's a lifelong problem and there is no cure of this problem till date. Some of the medications are used to reduce its symptoms and controlling it but these medications cannot be used to completely cure this problem.[4]

Therefore, early detection of the syndrome is very important to control its symptoms in the early stages. However, there is no medically defined test to specifically detect PCOS. Doctors have to take several different tests to detect the syndrome such as hormone test, blood test, pelvic ultrasound, and also have to rely on physical exam and appeared symptoms. Physicians give more significance to ultrasonography. But manual sonography can give wrong prediction. Manual prediction is also very time-consuming and misleads the diagnosis.[5]

Earlier research has been done on the ultrasound images to check the follicles count in the ovary using image classification and segmentation using machine learning techniques. Machine learning plays a crucial role in the detection and prediction of diseases in the bio-medical field such as cancer and diabetes. Majorly supervised learning is used for classification in medical field. Basically, in this, the model is trained using labeled data having correct detection and later the classification is done by the trained machine.[6]

Particle swarm optimization is done on segmented follicles to help in detection. Model based on F3I feature selection was used to detect follicles in enlarged ovaries.[7] Genes also play a crucial role in prediction. PCOS classification is also done using convolutional neural networks (CNNs) on ultrasound images to classify class as PCOS or non-PCOS using automated feature extraction.[8] In many cases, patient doesn't have cyst but shown infertility symptoms of PCOS due to genetic factors and PCOS history in the family. Lifestyle changes, diet, and mental health issues such as stress are also linked to PCOS. Cyst in the follicle alone cannot detect the PCOS. So afterward PCOS classification was also done on other clinical parameters by applying machine learning algorithm. Machine learning classification techniques used in research works were using logistic regression (LR) and Bayesian classifier to detect polycystic ovarian syndrome in automated screening.[9] Later on, a critical study was done focusing on the classification considering the feature selection and using naïve base classifiers, ID3 algorithm, and support vector machine (SVM) to find the highest accuracy among the classification algorithms.[14] Other research work was done using *K*-nearest neighbors (KNN) and random forest to calculate the mean absolute error. The binary classification is used to classify between two classes, that is, belongs to one class or to other but not both. This study focuses on analyzing and evaluating the clinical parameters playing a major role to detect the PCOS in women.[15]

5.2 LITERATURE SURVEY

PCOS has garnered the interest of many researchers and thus various methodologies and techniques have been proposed in the past to early detection and treatment of this disease. In this section, we have discussed some of the key findings and literature on PCOS detection based on machine learning techniques.

Bharati et al.[6] have shown the use of gradient boosting and hybrid of random forest and logistic regression for classification, taking 10 symptoms of the disease. Holdout method and *k*-cross-fold validation are used for performance analyses of algorithm in which precision and accuracy of RFLR are highest.

Mehrotra et al.[9] proposed classification of PCOS based on an automated screening. Twelve features were selected and multivariate linear regression is applied on the selected features. Bayesian classifier is used for the prediction over same data. This study shows that Bayesian classifier is better for detection of PCOS over LR.

Purnama et al.[16] proposed a system for classification on ultrasound images of ovaries. Gaussian-based filter is used in preprocessing to eliminate the noise from the images. Then contrast increment, binarization of images followed by edge detection and follicle cropping in segmentation. The work used neural network-learning vector quantization, KNN Euclidean distance test, and SVM for classification.

Meena et al.[14] classified PCOS on the basis of two machine learning algorithms J48 and ID3 and then they proposed the technique neural fuzzy rough set (NFRS) evaluation and used the information gain subset evaluation technique to get better accuracy. Meena et al.[15] proposed a feature selection method which is hybrid of artificial neural network (ANN) and NFRS. The attributes selected by NFRS are fed into the ANN algorithm which is used in the classification of PCOS. The use of hybrid feature selection gives high accuracy than many classification algorithms.

Wisesty et al.[19] proposed a method in which ultrasonographic images of ovaries are taken as input. Gray scaling is used in preprocessing followed by filtering and cleaning of data. The output of preprocessed data is later on used in feature selection using Gabor Wavelet and modification is done on backpropagation algorithms. Then, the modified version of algorithm was used to classify the data, IF.

The study of Sawant et al.[3] describes numerous effects of PCOS and drawn a comparison of treatment in different medical fields according to the symptoms. Cahyono et al.[8] proposed a system to classify ultrasound images of ovaries by using deep learning. CNN is used for proposed system consisting six layers, out of which two layers are convolutional layers. Visualization of ultrasound image at each layer is also shown to describe the process.

Soni et al.[17] have explored various risks related to cyst in ovaries and various data-mining techniques such as data classification, association rule mining clustering, and outlier detection that can be applied in the diagnosis of disease. Thufailah et al.[18] proposed a method for classification of PCOS based on the image classification of ultrasound images. Elman neural network was used for classification and then hidden layer test is done on the trained data and the tested data to check the accuracy. Zhang et al.[20] have exploited Raman spectroscopy on fluid of follicles and plasma. Result of PCA on Raman spectra has shown valuable differences between patients suffering with PCOS and non-PCOS patients.

Denny et al.[10] have proposed a system named i-HOPE. Machine learning classification algorithms are applied considering eight parameters related to metabolism and ultrasound images using PCA. They concluded that the random forest (RF) classifier gives more accuracy in differentiating PCOS patients and non-PCOS patient.

The work of Inan et al.[12] used chi-square test with feature selection. Synthetic minority oversampling and edited nearest neighbors were exploited to improve the selection of features to support ensemble learning model extreme gradient boosting (XGB).

5.3 FRAMEWORK FOR PCOS DETECTION

Adopting an efficient methodology is important for the efficient prediction of PCOS and hence many researches have considered machine learning algorithms for classifying the data as PCOS and non-PCOS. For the implementation of ML algorithms, initial cleaning and preprocessing of dataset is the fundamental requirement. Thus, this section deals with the basic steps and their details of preparation of dataset and the models selected for the comparison for PCOS classification. Following are the major steps employed for developing and tuning the appropriate machine learning models used in the classification of PCOS patients.

5.3.1 DATA COLLECTION

Collection of data is a crucial step which plays an important role in machine learning models. There are various sources from where dataset can be taken like UCL and Kaggle. Dataset of PCOS patients has been taken from Kaggle repository (https://www.kaggle.com/prasoonkottarathil/polycystic-ovary-syndrome-pcos). It contains 541 rows and 44 columns including the target column containing information about whether the patient suffers from disease if numerical data is 1 (yes) or does not suffer if the numerical data is 0 (no). The dataset contains biological and physical parameters that can be used for PCOS prediction.

5.3.2 DATA PREPROCESSING

The data are preprocessed before passing it as input for the machine learning models. Preprocessing is important as the output of the model depends upon the input given to the models. This process includes handling of any missing data if exists as machine learning models are unable to read missing data. Data have to be divided for the testing and training purpose for validation and verification of the machine learning model proposed. The splitting of dataset is done randomly based on the type of algorithm selected. Most commonly, the split ratio is taken as 8:2, that is, 80% of data are used for training the model and 20% of data are used for testing the model. In this study of ML techniques proposed for PCOS detection also, we have considered the same data distribution for all the models.

TABLE 5.1 List of Parameters.

	Numeric-based parameters		String-based parameters
PCOS	No. of abortions	PRL (ng/ml)	Marriage status (Y/N)
Age (years)	I beta HCG (hb/ml)	Vit D3	Pregnant
Weight	II beta HCG (hb/ml)	PRG (ng/ml)	Weight gain (Y/N)
Height	FSH (mlU/ml)	RBS (mg/dl)	Hair growth (Y/N)
BMI	LH (mlU/ml)	BP_Systolic (mmHg)	Skin darkening (Y/N)
Blood group	FSH/LH	BP_Diastolic (mmHg)	Hair loss (Y/N)
Pulse rate	Hip (in)	Follicle no. (L)	Pimples (Y/N)
RR	Waist (in)	Follicle no. (R)	Fast food (Y/N)
Hb	Waist:hip ratio	Avg. *F* size (L) (mm)	Regular exercise (Y/N)
Cycle	TSH (mIU/l)	Avg. *F* size (R) (mm)	
Cycle length	AMH (ng/ml)	Endocardium (mm)	

5.3.3 FEATURE SELECTION

After data preprocessing, the next important step is selection of features on the basis of which the prediction is supposed to be done. To remove the irrelevant and avoid redundant features from the dataset, relevant features are selected based on their correlation with PCOS. One of the methods to do so is to use correlation matrix that shows the correlation of each feature with target column. Correlation matrix's lower triangular portion is mirror image of the upper triangular portion and correlation values vary from −1 to 1. These values show the relation between two features. Diagonal of the matrix always gives 1 as value because each feature horizontally shows correlation with itself. Features having correlation value higher than 0.4 are selected which include follicle no. (R), follicle no. (L), skin darkening, hair growth, weight gain, and cycle.

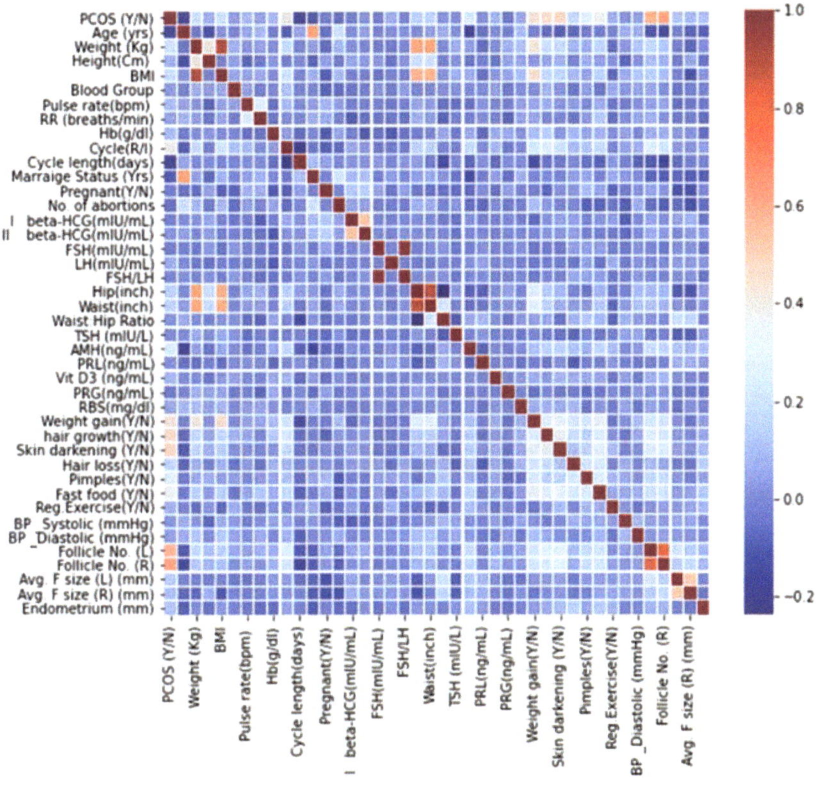

FIGURE 5.1 Correlation matrix.

5.3.4 EVALUATION METRICS

To investigate the performance of the technique proposed and its efficacy compared to other methods in the literature, evaluation metrics are used to measure the effectiveness of the method proposed. Following metrics are commonly used by research community to evaluate the success of the technique:

Accuracy: It is the proportion of correct predictions to that of total predictions made, which is computed as

$$\text{Accuracy} = \frac{\text{TP} + \text{TN}}{\text{TP} + \text{TN} + \text{FP} + \text{FN}} \tag{5.1}$$

Precision: It is the ratio of true positives to sum of true positives and false positives, calculated as

$$\text{Precision} = \frac{\text{TP}}{\text{TP} + \text{FP}} \tag{5.2}$$

Recall: It is the ratio of true positives to sum of true positives and false negatives, given by

$$\text{Recall} = \frac{\text{TP}}{\text{TP} + \text{FN}} \tag{5.3}$$

F1_score: It is the harmonic mean of precision and recall and gives a measure of incorrectly classified cases.

$$\text{F1\_score} = 2 \times \frac{\text{Precision} \times \text{Recall}}{\text{Precision} + \text{Recall}} \tag{5.4}$$

where TP stands for true positives, TN stands for true negatives, FP stands for false positives, and FN stands for false negatives.

5.4 STATE-OF-THE-ART TECHNIQUES

This section discusses the majorly adopted state-of-the-art machine learning techniques for PCOS diagnostics.

Logistic regression (LR): LR is a machine learning algorithm used for classification and regression. It uses sigmoidal function because sigmoidal function squishes the value either toward the top margin, that is, 1, or toward the bottom margin, that is, 0. So, the output can belong to either of the categories. The output of the LR is also a form of log odds as in deriving the equation; log of odds is taken.[9]

Gaussian-naïve Bayes (Gaussian NB): Naïve Bayes is the classification algorithm based on the Bayes theorem. It describes the probability of an event based on the conditions known that might be related to the event. An assumption is made that the presence of a feature in a class is independent of other features present. Even if the features are correlated or dependent on each other, then also all the properties contribute independently. That is why, it is also called naïve.[6]

K-nearest neighbor (KNN): It is a supervised learning algorithm mostly used for classification. It is based on the similarities among the available cases and the new input case. It searches for the *K* similar instances and classifies the new input to the instance with which it has the most similarity.[13]

Decision tree (DT): This is a type of supervised learning in which the algorithm uses tree representation for the classification and prediction. An assumption is made that the whole training set will be considered as the root of the tree. On the basis of the value of attributes, the dataset is distributed in recursive manner. The leaf nodes are the target columns and the internal nodes represent the attributes.

Random forest (RF): It is a supervised learning algorithm and an ensemble of multiple DTs. It is best used for classification and also avoids the problem of overfitting. Each DT selects the random set of rows as input in the dataset and predicts the output. The majority voting of the resulted output from these DTs gives the final result of classification.[11]

Xtreme gradient boosting (XGB): Extreme gradient boosting is a part of ensemble learning. Gradient boosting employs gradient descent algorithm to minimize errors in sequential model. The model is optimized using an arbitrarily differentiable function and an optimization algorithm.[12]

5.5 COMPARATIVE RESULTS AND DISCUSSION

For an experimental study of various abovementioned techniques, a total record of 541 patients having 541 rows and 44 columns were considered for implementation. For performance analysis, evaluation measures such as accuracy, precision, recall, and F1_score are taken as metrics to compare these chosen techniques.[14]

For LR, the accuracy obtained is 87.04% with precision of 82.50% and F1_score 82.50%.

For Gaussian NB, the accuracy obtained is 84.26% and recall percentage is 85.0%. Precision and F1_score percentage for naïve Bayes is 75.56 and 80.0%, respectively.

Results for K-NN showed the accuracy of 63.89%, with precision 52.17% and recall as 30%, along with the F1_score percentage of 38.10%. RF gave an accuracy of 86.11%, a precision percentage 87.88%, recall percentage 72.50%, and F1_score percentage 79.45%.

Resultant of Decision Tree Classifier has an accuracy percentage of 83.33%, precision value 77.50%, recall value 77.50%, and F1_score of 77.50%.

XG boost classification has shown accuracy percentage of 90.74%, precision of 87.50%, recall value 87.50%, and F1_score percentage of 87.50%.

Figure 5.2 shows the performance based on ROC curves of LR, Gaussian NB, RF, K-NN, DT, and XGB classifiers.

Figures 5.3 and 5.4 show the comparative analysis of six compared techniques (LR, Gaussian NB, KNN, RF, DT, and XGB), based on aforementioned evaluation metrics (accuracy, precision, recall, and F1_score).

Overall, among all the state-of-the-art techniques compared, XG boost gives the best result for classification of this syndrome followed by LR and then RF classification.

TABLE 5.2 Quantitative Analysis of State-of-the-Art Classifiers.

Algorithm	Accuracy (%)	Precision (%)	Recall (%)	F1 score (%)
KNN	63.89	52.17	30.00	38.10
DT	83.33	77.50	77.50	77.50
Gaussian NB	84.26	75.56	85.00	80.00
RF	86.11	**87.88**	72.50	79.45
LR	87.04	82.50	82.50	82.50
XGB	**90.74**	87.50	**87.50**	87.50

5.6 CONCLUSION

PCOS is a most common condition among women nowadays which can become worse if not dealt properly in the initial age and can have severe symptoms and side effects. After being a prevalent syndrome, still the root cause of this syndrome is not found by medical practitioners. But there are many biological and clinical parameters that are useful in its diagnosis. This chapter has dealt with certain selected clinical parameters that are found to be contributing the most in the diagnosis and drawn a comparison of various machine learning models that are used for the classification of PCOS patients. Total six parameters, follicle no. (R), follicle no. (L), skin darkening, hair growth, weight gain, and cycle, are taken into consideration from the 41 available features on the basis of their correlation with the PCOS. A total of 541 patient records were fitted into different machine learning algorithms including LR, Gaussian naïve Bayes classification, KNN, RF Classification, DT, and XGB algorithm. Out of all selected algorithms, XG boost outperforms the rest of the algorithms. LR performed the second best followed by RF algorithm, Gaussian Naïve Bayes, DT, and KNN. As of future work, the accuracy obtained can be increased by developing hybrid classification models and the models can also be applied on a much larger dataset of patients.

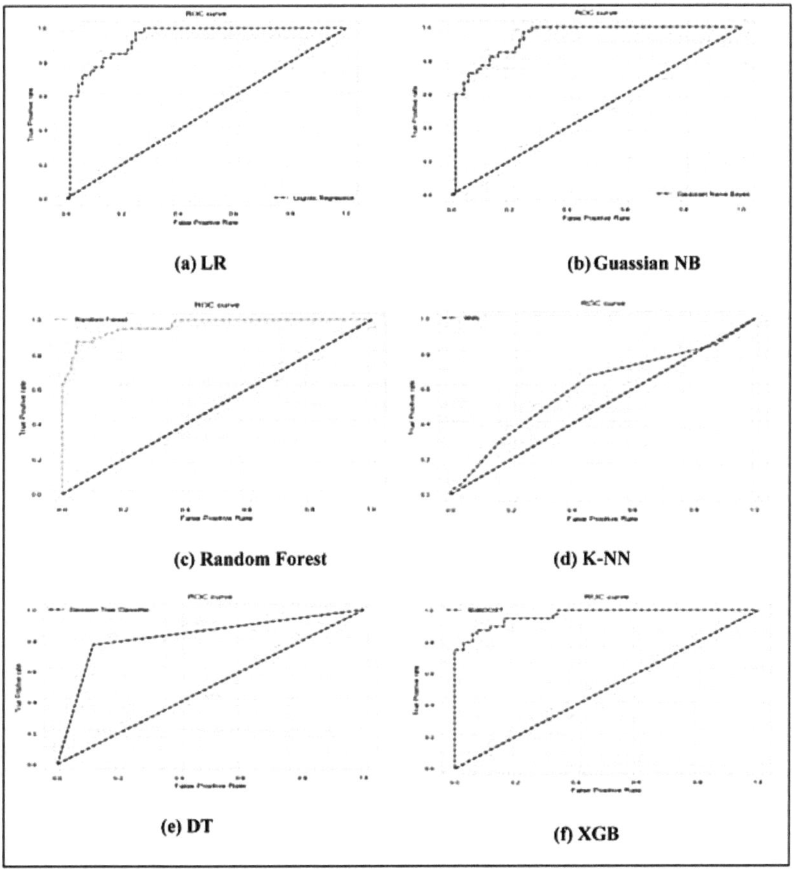

FIGURE 5.2 ROC curves of state-of-the-art classifiers. (a) LR; (b) Gaussian NB; (c) random forest; (d) KNN; (e) DT; and (f) (XGB).

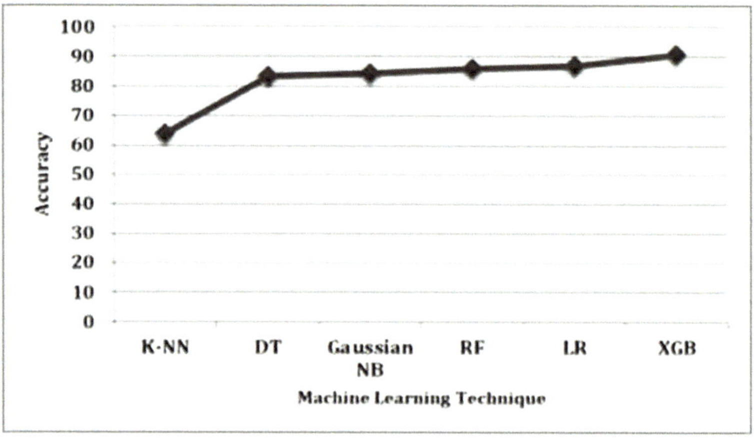

FIGURE 5.3 Performance comparison based on accuracy.

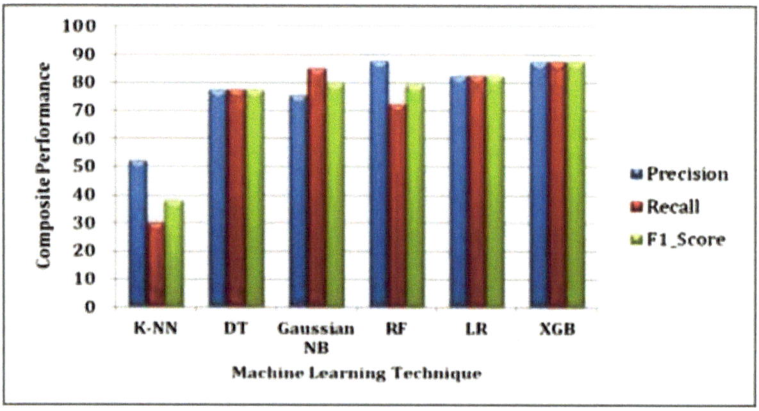

FIGURE 5.4 Comparative analysis of techniques based on precision, recall, and F1_score.

KEYWORDS

- **PCOS**
- **machine learning**
- **supervised classification**
- **polycystic ovary syndrome**

REFERENCES

1. Bremer, A. A. Polycystic Ovary Syndrome in the Pediatric Population. *Metab. Syndr. Relat. Disorders* **2010,** *8* (5), 375–394.
2. March, W. A.; Moore, V. M.; Willson, K. J.; Phillips, D. I.; Norman, R. J.; Davies, M. J. The Prevalence of Polycystic Ovary Syndrome in a Community Sample Assessed under Contrasting Diagnostic Criteria. *Hum. Reprod.* **2010,** 25(2), 544–551.
3. Sawant, A.; Patil, S.; Shah, S. Review on PCOD/PCOS & Its Treatment in Different Medicinal Systems—Allopathy, Ayurveda, Homeopathy. *Sci. J.* **2017,** *1*(1), 1–16.
4. Okoroh, E. M.; Hooper, W. C.; Atrash, H. K.; Yusuf, H. R.; Boulet, S. L. Prevalence of Polycystic Ovary Syndrome among the Privately Insured, United States, 2003–2008. *Am. J. Obstetr. Gynecol.* **2012,** 207(4), 299-e1.
5. Priya, N.; Jeevitha, S. Overview of an Ovarian Classification and Detection PCOS in Ultrasound Image: A Study. In *International Conference on Information, Communication and Computing Technology*; Springer: Cham, 2019; pp 359–365.
6. Bharati, S.; Podder, P.; Mondal, M. R. H. Diagnosis of Polycystic Ovary Syndrome Using Machine Learning Algorithms. In *2020 IEEE Region 10 Symposium (TENSYMP)*; IEEE: New York, NY, 2020; pp 1486–1489.
7. Setiawati, E.; Tjokorda, A. B. W. Particle Swarm Optimization on Follicles Segmentation to Support PCOS Detection. In *2015 3rd International Conference on Information and Communication Technology (ICoICT)*; IEEE: New York, NY, 2015; pp 369–374.
8. Cahyono, B.; Mubarok, M. S.; Wisesty, U. N. An Implementation of Convolutional Neural Network on PCO Classification Based on Ultrasound Image. In *2017 5th International Conference on Information and Communication Technology (ICoIC7)*; IEEE: New York, NY, 2017; pp 1–4.
9. Mehrotra, P.; Chatterjee, J.; Chakraborty, C.; Ghoshdastidar, B.; Ghoshdastidar, S. Automated Screening of Polycystic Ovary Syndrome Using Machine Learning Techniques. In *2011 Annual IEEE India Conference*; IEEE: New York, NY, 2011; pp 1–5.
10. Denny, A.; Raj, A.; Ashok, A.; Ram, C. M.; George, R. i-HOPE: Detection and Prediction System for Polycystic Ovary Syndrome (PCOS) Using Machine Learning Techniques. In *TENCON 2019–2019 IEEE Region 10 Conference (TENCON)*; IEEE: New York, NY, 2019; pp. 673–678.
11. Hassan, M. M.; Mirza, T. Comparative Analysis of Machine Learning Algorithms in Diagnosis of Polycystic Ovarian Syndrome. *Int. J. Comput. Appl.* **2020,** *975*, 8887.
12. Inan, M. S. K.; Ulfath, R. E.; Alam, F. I.; Bappee, F. K.; Hasan, R. Improved Sampling and Feature Selection to Support Extreme Gradient Boosting for PCOS Diagnosis. In *2021 IEEE 11th Annual Computing and Communication Workshop and Conference (CCWC)*; IEEE: New York, NY, 2021; pp 1046–1050.
13. Legro, R. S.; Arslanian, S. A.; Ehrmann, D. A.; Hoeger, K. M.; Murad, M. H.; Pasquali, R.; Welt, C. K. Diagnosis and Treatment of Polycystic Ovary Syndrome: An Endocrine Society Clinical Practice Guideline. *J. Clin. Endocrinol. Metab.* **2013,** *98* (12), 4565–4592.
14. Meena, D. K.; Manimekalai, D. M.; Rethinavalli, S. A Novel Framework for Filtering the PCOS Attributes Using Data Mining Techniques. *Int. J. Eng. Res. Technol.* **2015,** *4*(1), 702–706.

15. Meena, K.; Manimekalai, M.; Rethinavalli, S. Correlation of Artificial Neural Network Classification and NFRS Attribute Filtering Algorithm for PCOS Data. *Int. J. Res. Eng. Technol.* **2015,** *4*(3), 519–524.
16. Purnama, B.; Wisesti, U. N.; Nhita, F.; Gayatri, A.; Mutiah, T. A Classification of Polycystic Ovary Syndrome Based on Follicle Detection of Ultrasound Images. In *2015 3rd International Conference on Information and Communication Technology (ICoICT)*; IEEE: New York, NY, 2015; pp 396–401.
17. Soni, P.; Vashisht, S. Exploration on Polycystic Ovarian Syndrome and Data Mining Techniques. In *2018 3rd International Conference on Communication and Electronics Systems (ICCES)*; IEEE: New York, NY, 2018, pp 816–820.
18. Thufailah, I. F.; Wisesty, U. N. An Implementation of Elman Neural Network for Polycystic Ovary Classification Based on Ultrasound Images. *J. Phys.: Conf. Ser.* **2018,** *971* (1), 012016.
19. Wisesty, U. N.; Nasri, J. Modified Backpropagation Algorithm for Polycystic Ovary Syndrome Detection Based on Ultrasound Images. In *International Conference on Soft Computing and Data Mining*. Springer: Cham, 2016; pp 141–151.
20. Zhang, X.; Liang, B.; Zhang, J.; Hao, X.; Xu, X.; Chang, H. M.; Tan, J. Raman Spectroscopy of Follicular Fluid and Plasma with Machine-Learning Algorithms for Polycystic Ovary Syndrome Screening. *Mol. Cell. Endocrinol.* **2021,** *523*, 111139.

CHAPTER 6

A Comprehensive Review on Diagnosis of Alzheimer's Disease Using Ensemble Methods and Machine Learning

PRACHI PATIL and SUJATA KADU

Terna Engineering College, Navi Mumbai, India

ABSTRACT

Alzheimer's illness is one of the most common diseases on the planet that is responsible to increase the number of death rate among the elderly populace. This illness is considered to occur due to a brain disorder that results in the malfunctioning of an individual's thinking and reading ability. According to the statistics, approximately 40 million people across the globe have been victimized over this disease. However, the root cause of this disease happens to be dementia, which disconnects the nerve cells in the brain, eventually resulting in memory lapse. Despite the fact of advanced technology, the human race still lacks the prevention of this disease. Hence, the doctors came up with a solution for detecting the disease in the earlier stages so that the process of memory lapse can be slowed down. Therefore, the discernment of Alzheimer's in the earlier stages became a crucial part of the health-care industry. In times where early detection of this illness could solve the issue, scientists came up with machine learning (ML). ML is a subcategory of Artificial Intelligence that works on the fundamentals of optimization techniques over complex datasets. Further, the concept of ML was extended to detect and diagnose

Applied Intelligence for Medical Image Analysis. Aarti, Raju Pal, Mukesh Saraswat, & Himanshu Mittal (Eds.)

a multiple variety of other diseases as well. As a result, the author of this research tends to put forward the contribution of ML in diagnosing Alzheimer's in the premature stages. In the current study, surveys on the existing ML techniques along with a combination of ensemble methods are reviewed.

6.1 INTRODUCTION

The doctors generally refer to this disease as a neurological brain disorder that causes the nerve cells to not function as they should in an ideal case. This disease is meant to increase over time and is sometimes known as slow progression illness. Hence, the doctors categorize it into initial symptoms and advanced-stage symptoms. Memory loss is expected to be the target of the person in the early phases as he tends to undergo relapse. These symptoms then further move into the advanced stage where the illness is considered to take a serious turn. All these signs happen to affect and change a person's emotional, physical, and mental capabilities. Unfortunately, there still doesn't exist an accurate cure for this disease, although the symptoms of a patient can be very well worked upon and treated. However, these treatments are not meant to cure the patient or remove the illness, rather their purpose is to temporarily reduce the aftereffects of the illness. Therefore, it is said that the earlier a person is diagnosed with the disease, the more are its chances to receive treatment. Further, this kind of treatment is proposed by the fundamentals of machine learning (ML) that allows computers and machines to learn by themselves with little or minimal human intervention.[1] Based on this set of information, the machine tends to predict, diagnose, and establish relationships to give the desired output.[2] This is one of the major reasons that this field is being explored to attain maximum efficiency and profit due to its precise impact in classifying and detecting an illness. Hence, this concept is observed to increase exponentially in the field of medicine to its maximum potential. Despite the number of advantages this concept offers, researchers are still unable to find the best match of algorithms and techniques to detect the same. For example, a study involving multiple facets of ML acquired an accuracy of 80%,[3] although it was well aware of the parameters used to detect the same. It however failed to increase the accuracy from 80% to a little more using other ML algorithms.[4] In situations where the researchers need to decide which element of feature extraction should fit where, a challenging task in dementia detection remains. Despite the fact that a lot of health-care industries have already made their equipment built-in with ML, the challenge of using which technique and algorithm where still happens to be a difficult task.[5] The process of drug discovery in the medical field first involves the selection of a supervised learning algorithm and feature extraction techniques to further infiltrate the procedure and take the project to a more latter stage. This procedure of extracting the right amount of information and knowledge at the right time helps to diagnose any previously unseen or future experiences.[6,7] However, in every scenario, the nature of input data determines how the software would function. Hence, this part validates a significant character in regulating the performance of techniques and algorithms used. Researchers have witnessed that some model-derived algorithms work exceptionally well with standardized data,[8] whereas on the other hand, a combination of algorithms and techniques under ML works exceptionally well on regulated and unstandardized data.[9] Thus, the authors of this research suggest that the selection of algorithm validates a vital role in discovering the performance of the resulted framework. Hence, this chapter exemplifies a comparative survey among ML methods and ensemble methods. The combination of ML methods put forward in this chapter are logistic regression (LR), naive Bayes (NB), *k*-nearest neighbors (KNN), random forest (RF), decision tree (DT), multilayer perceptron (MLP), and support vector machines (SVM), followed by ensemble methods that are gradient boosting and XGBoost.

Following are the objectives of the proposed study:

- To go through multiple research papers based on the related domain.
- To conduct a comparative analysis of the existing methods and convey it through a table.
- To analyze what parameters can be used to detect the disease so that maximum accuracy can be achieved.
- To conduct a review based on ML and ensemble learning methods.

This entire survey chapter is distributed into three sections: an introduction, followed by the literature review, carried out to understand different ML algorithm and ensemble learning methods. To summarize the research carried out in this chapter, conclusion has been drawn.

6.2 LITERATURE REVIEW

As mentioned above, this disease does not possess a cure but can only be treated once it is brought to the notice of the doctor. Therefore, it is said that only an early detection might help to recover this illness. In one of the reports, it has been brought to witness that by 2050 almost one-third of the population shall be victimized by this disease and almost 1 in every 80 individuals might suffer from Alzheimer's. In a study by Reynolds,[10] the authors proposed the use of the Gaussian mixer model (GMM) that could detect AD-based MR images and further classify the disease. The GMM algorithm successfully extracted all the required features and later performed a dimensionality reduction process to enhance the accuracy of the overall system. The same concept of the GMM model was also used by Bui and Hoang,[11] wherein the fundamentals of the Bayesian network were also brought in and combined for execution purposes. This developed model was later compared with multiple other conventional following models and algorithms such as SVM and KNN. Thus, precise diagnosis is the only way to end this disease in the early stages through the usage of ML. Furthermore, this concept is capable of not only detecting the disease but also classifying it under a category marked. The exceptional quality of this concept is that the machine tends to perform all of its execution just by the knowledge fed to it during the input stage and generally happens to outperform other routine algorithms. This is one of the major reasons that ML is used in the medical field to detect, diagnose, and classify the requested disease based on image forming, retrieval, and storage. This contribution has helped to increase the potential in the field of radiology, where X-rays and CT images are used. In another work by Armananzas et al.,[12] the authors proposed the diagnosis of AD disease using MR images that could further classify the disease and prevent its occurrence in the later stages. In Zhu et al.,[13] functional MR images were predominantly used and statistical maps were determined using a parametric mapping toolbox. The voxels from the toolbox[14] were selected using filters and a ranking scheme was developed. In another study by Lahmiri and Boukadoum,[15] a novel method was proposed by authors that could detect the presence of the disease by modeling MR images as fractal objects. In the same model, the method of feature extraction was used using Hurst's exponents along with SVM classifiers. In the later stages, the model was able to distinguish AD from healthy people and mild cognitive impairment (MCI)-related patients. When the same experiment was carried out in the later stages, the model showed high levels of accuracy. Therefore, the authors believe that the dataset available to predict AD is comparatively small with regards to the amount of research that is required to predict the same. However, recent modalities and high outturn prognostics have left us with significant calculations of epithelial, pharmacological, and microbiological guidelines to manage. As in today's world, standard metrics and basic instincts do not always work. The use of ML in disease prediction and visualization is part of a larger trend toward foresight and personalized treatment. In Srinivasan et al.,[16] the authors used the concept of discrete wavelet transform with the images of fractal features. In this model, the initial steps involved image processing and feature extraction. A four-classification technique was further carried out and results were analyzed based on the performance analysis. The model tends to accomplish an overall accuracy of 89.7%. In a research work by Zheng et al.,[17] the authors proposed an algorithm involving the concepts of Boltzmann classification. The model used SVM as classifiers and further classified multimodal data. The model was combined with the concepts of RBM and SVM in the later stages.

This shift is significant not only for patients seeking to improve their lifestyles but also for clinicians seeking medical resolutions and health analysts. Before delving into the specifics of ML methods, it is important to first comprehend what ML is and what ML systems are typically used in Alzheimer's disease prognosis. ML is a subset of artificial intelligence that includes a variety of tools for applying quantitative, stochastic decisions based on prior learning. It employs prior knowledge (training) to label new events and forecast future patterns. ML is far more powerful than traditional statistical techniques. To achieve effective results in ML, complete knowledge of the problem and the restrictions of the algorithms are required. As a result, if experimentation is conducted properly, training is cautiously applied, and outcomes are strongly referenced, it has a good chance of success. Furthermore, all of the models and techniques used in ML are somewhat unique. For example, some methods are established based on certain hypotheses or for a particular dataset, rendering them inapplicable to other types of data. That is why it is critical to use multiple ML methods on the same training data.

A detailed study on the classification of AD has been put forward by many analysts. In this section, all methods and materials, block diagrams, and research work related to the algorithm used are discussed below.

6.2.1 MACHINE LEARNING ALGORITHMS

ML generally has three kinds of learning algorithms: supervised learning, unsupervised learning, and reinforcement learning. In supervised learning, learning data are provided and the program attempts to learn it by drawing the input to the desired output. Self-learning is used by unsupervised learning algorithms on unclassified and unlabeled data. SVM, AR mining, and ensemble methods are also commonly used techniques. In comparison to the preceding techniques, SVM, or SVM, is somewhat newer technique that is now a well-known ML technique, but it is virtually unknown in the field of prognosis.

6.2.1.1 SUPPORT VECTOR MACHINE

As mentioned earlier, the researchers make use of a combination of algorithms and methods to conclude certain disease detections. In Rabeh et al.,[18] the authors made use of two algorithms under ML: SVM and DTs. In this study, the researchers analyzed three parts of the brain, mainly, frontal, sagittal, and axial. The entire implementation took place on the OASIS database that was based on MRI images of a person suffering from Alzheimer's. Where the detection of the disease was done using SVM, the final classification was achieved using DTs. In this case, the parameters used to classify were considered to be hippocampus, corpus callosum, and cortex.

The difference between Alzheimer's and other diseases is that Alzheimer's tends to increase gradually in an individual after hitting a certain age, unlike dementia that happens to grow from infancy. However, both diseases are responsible for memory loss in its own way. The disease is classified into three groups on the basis of its infection on the left and right hemispheres. In individuals that are prone to weakness, the enfolding of this disease initiates on the hippocampus and frontal cortex of the brain tissues. Further, the disease tends to expand to the bottom and side portions of the cortex. Burbidge et al.[19] demonstrated that the SVM classification model has the potential to be used for framework analysis method. They conducted a benchmark test in which they equated SVM to different classifiers currently in use in this field. It was known that this process could predict the presence of dihydrofolate in brain tissues. Further, the testing was carried out on ANN, and the authors concluded that SVM performed better than any of the known and experimented methods.

In Valentini,[20] the analysts suggested a technique based on the concepts of SVM combined with Gaussian kernels. It was observed that this method proved to give better efficiency to distinguish normal tissues from those of malignant tissues and investigate the role of sets of coordinately expressed genes in lymphoid tissue carcinogenesis. Using gene expression data from the "Lymphochip," he demonstrated that SVM can accurately differentiate tumoral tissues and that OC ensembles can effectively identify multiple kinds of lymphoma. Li et al.[21] used SVMs to categorize texture using translation-invariant feature extraction, taking DWFT as input. To further diminish the issue of selecting appropriate values for kernel, the researchers put forward a concept based on fusion schemes.

6.2.1.2 DECISION TREES

In Saputra et al.,[22] the authors used a combination of DTs along with particle swarm optimization (PSO) algorithm. The dataset used was taken from Kaggle repository named as OASIS 2. The authors implemented the concept with 10-fold cross-validation. Feature selection is performed using the algorithm and an accuracy of 91.15% is obtained. This study desires to focus AD using the dataset obtained from Kaggle repository. Further, it tends to obtain the best precision values by combining it with PSO algorithm based on DTs. It was however observed that the algorithm worked better when performed along with PSO algorithm.

The process flow of the entire DT model is depicted in the figure above. The same approach is used in the DT model. The model was trained without being fine-tuned, and then the grid search was used to find the best model parameters to fine-tune the model. In this case, the PSO measure has been examined to evaluate the tree's standard, and a scope has been chosen to evaluate the tree's depth. It decides on each node and goes into greater detail. It predicts the best solution after analyzing all of the node choices.

Because PSO can optimize datasets and select only those attribute features that would have an effective response on the DT algorithm. DT classification is a traditional data classification technique that has a wide range of applications. DTs can be built in a variety of ways as branch-like fragments. To improve the order of execution, Bi et al.[23] proposed the random neural system group. The Alzheimer's disease neuroimaging initiative provided the dataset for their experiment (ADNI). With 92.31% accuracy, the Elman Neural Network was confirmed to be an ideal base classifier that utilizes the arbitrary neural system cluster that is dependent on the outcome of highlighted selections. Bi et al.[24] used the random SVM clustering approach to characterize AD and group the disease with 92.31% accuracy. Joshi et al.[25] used various ML techniques, including multilayer neural networks, to develop multiple frameworks for the identification of AD.

6.2.1.3 LOGISTIC REGRESSION

The fundamentals of LR are deeply rooted between features and log classes that tend to be linear. In simple words, the probability of each class happens to be a sigmoid function to a feature vector. Later n number of parameters are calculated for every independent class and simultaneously a score corresponding to each data point x is calculated. In Piers et al.,[26] authors used the concept of LR along with genetic algorithm (GA) to detect and classify the disease. This suggested theory depicts the ability of GA in the field of neural science. It demonstrated that combining a specific selection of variables outperforms using all of the single significant variables in the system for chronic disease prediction. However, the variables that are selected by GA happen to be a more important aspect of the entire algorithm.

The LR model, like the SVM, has been approached in the same way. It identifies the variables that are independent and dependent. It makes use of the sigmoid function to forecast probabilities and set decision boundaries. Ebadi et al.[27] also implemented a classification model by combining various machine learning models (such as LR, RF, NB, KNN, and SVM). This model also tested a k-best feature selection method where the features were ranked based on their power of efficiency and performance. This method was able to classify AD patients with an overall accuracy of 80%.

6.2.1.4 RANDOM FOREST

ML characterization has been one of the widely accepted advancement in recent years. In many scientific fields, the RF technique has been successfully used to reduce high-dimensional and multi-source statistics. The primary goal is to investigate the current state of the art in the use of RF dual-brain images for the identification of AD. The below block diagram depicts the whole RF model which generally remains the same while detecting the disease.

In a review by Sarica et al.,[28] the authors adopted the technique of RF to diagnose AD, wherein the majority of the attributes were derived from the ADNI dataset consisting of MRI images. In various studies, the model achieved an accuracy of 90% and 82% when it was being implemented using only RF algorithm and a combination of RF with SVM, respectively. On the other hand, a three-class classification was being performed on a dataset of AD versus MCI versus HC patients. This model achieved an accuracy of 53% and 96%, when it was implemented using RF alone and a blend of RF and KNN, respectively. Quite a similar amount of study is been suggested by Dimitriadis *et al.* that also includes a systematic review of ML strategies.[29] On the other hand, multiple surveys for diagnostic classification are also being provided by Rathore et al.[30–32]

6.2.1.5 KNN

In Dinu and Ganesan,[33] the authors combined the methods of LR along with KNN for AD diagnosis. In this method, they also used *T*-test method for the classification purpose. Since KNN happens to be one of the most widely accepted ML techniques, known for its ease of classification, the authors proposed to detect the severity of the disease using the same. This method is generally opted by researchers as it increases the efficiency to a much higher level by distinguishing the components of the dataset and categorizing them under vectors by considering their respective classes. This also results in reduced time interval for the entire procedure to be carried out. In Dinu and Ganesan,[33] authors worked on the dataset containing patient's information including details about normal, MCI, and AD. Initially, the input images of the brain are fed to the preprocessing unit that is responsible for disease analysis using minimal number of features.

Horn et al.[34] proposed his work by working upon 116 attributes of AD patients and performed his diagnosis on frontotemporal dementia. He carried out this experiment using classifiers (such as LDA, SVM, KNN, and MLP). These classifiers were used in various combinations to achieve the highest accuracy and finally the combination of KNN along with SVM was chosen as it gave an accuracy of 88% when performed together. On the other hand, ensemble techniques were also used to detect the same by multiple authors who worked using an MRI dataset of patients experiencing the same disease.[35] The algorithms so used were a combination of AdaBoost and Gaussian models. The overall accuracy reached was around 84.38%.

6.2.1.6 NAIVE BAYES

The naive Bayes classifies a testing dataset based on its attainable probability. It is quite unresponsive to oversampling. When it comes to reaching an equitable classifier model, NB is one of the best. It also has the greatest AUC. In Carnero-Pardo et al.,[36] the authors have focused on accuracy parameters of mainly two data sets: Euro test and photo test. In Williams et al.[37] and Schmitter-Edgecombe et al.,[38] authors have executed ML techniques to detect AD using NB, neural network, SVM, and DT.

6.2.1.7 MULTILAYER PERCEPTRON

The concept of neural networks is inspired from human neurons wherein the arrangement of these is similar to biological neural networks. It generally has two classifiers: input processing layer followed by an output layer. In MLP, the working of the input layer is similar to those of dendrites in human and that of output layer being similar to that of axons.

An MLP is a subcategory of ANN that functions as a feedforward network and has been recently used in many fields. This algorithm is a constructive algorithm for differentiating linear data. This algorithm is primarily used to detect and classify AD using arterial pulse transmission condition. Hence, this method is considered to be a supervised classifier. The feedforward function of this network works on backpropagation for training purpose. It generally comprises three consecutive layers followed as input, hidden, and output, respectively. The concept of this algorithm is put to use when no other algorithmic solution exists or in situations where the defined variables are too complex to be designed. However, this method is widely accepted in the fields of pattern recognition. Hence, its usage was derived to detect early presence of AD in a patient. This network also works on MRI images taken from imaging modalities.

6.2.2 ENSEMBLE LEARNING TECHNIQUES

Ensemble learning is a technique that combines multiple classifier problems and constructs a single set of base classifiers from it. The fundamentals of this technique are vitally based on voting and average weight classifiers. Several algorithms follow this concept of EL such boosting, bagging, and stacking. Based on which classifier model is to be used, EL divides it into two approaches, mainly heterogeneous and homogenous. The first approach is applied when multiple algorithms work on same set of training data, whereas the other algorithm works when same algorithm is applied on multiple training datasets. However, it is observed that both the frameworks significantly help in increasing the efficiency and robustness of a system. The overall contribution of the work is mentioned in Table 6.1 as the authors present a comparative analysis of the review so conducted.

6.2.2.1 ADABOOST

AdaBoost is an ensemble technique that is used to train trees by consecutively joining a series of weak classifiers. This chain of weak classifiers in turn tries to improve the entire network by handling the misclassified samples by previous classifiers. In this way, as a whole, the network seems to be categorized as a strong classifier. ML methods such as DTs are accompanied to reduce the issue of overfitting and are referred to as "stumps." Here, the DT is responsible to focus on the weaknesses of the previous tree and balance the entire weight. The accuracy of the network increases when more weak trees are added to it; however, this might result in overfitting problem.

6.2.2.2 GRADIENT BOOSTING

The concept of gradient boosting is used for classification models in order to forecast a model, similar to that of weak prediction models. This concept makes use of 1H-MRS biomarkers to predict AD among patients, which are then further used as a final classifier. The authors conducted experiments to evaluate and demonstrate the efficiency of the concept used.

TABLE 6.1 A Comparative Analysis of the Review So Conducted.

Ref.	Title	Domain	Concept	Dataset model	Output
[1]	Diagnosis of Alzheimer's disease in early step using SVM (support vector machine)	Machine learning	SVM + decision trees	OASIS	83% accuracy
[2]	Machines for pharmaceutical data analysis	Machine learning	SVM	ADNI	80% accuracy
[3]	Gene expression data analysis of human lymphoma using support vector machines and output coding ensembles	Machine learning	SVM + gene analysis	OASIS	87% accuracy
[4]	Texture classification using the support vector machines	Machine learning	SVM + DWFT	Brodatz	92% accuracy
[5]	Detecting Alzheimer's disease by the decision tree methods based on particle swarm optimization	Machine learning	SVM + decision trees	OASIS	95% accuracy
[6]	Random support vector machine cluster analysis of resting-state fMRI in Alzheimer's disease	Machine learning	SVM + Gaussian network	ADNI	95.48% accuracy
[7]	Classification and treatment of different stages of Alzheimer's disease using various machine learning methods	Machine learning	KNN + decision trees	ADNI	92.83% accuracy
[8]	Automated detection of brain atrophy patterns based on MRI for the prediction of Alzheimer's disease	Machine learning	SVM + random forest	OASIS	92.75% accuracy
[9]	Genetic algorithm with logistic regression for prediction of progression to Alzheimer's disease	Machine learning	Logistic regression + genetic algorithm	ADNI	93.56% accuracy
[10]	Random forest algorithm for the classification of neuroimaging data in Alzheimer's disease: a systematic review. frontiers in aging	Machine learning	Random forest + KNN	OASIS	90.52% accuracy
[11]	Multivariate data analysis and machine learning in Alzheimer's disease with a focus on structural magnetic resonance imaging	Machine learning	KNN + logistic regression	OASIS	95.63% accuracy
[12]	Automated diagnosis of Alzheimer's disease with degenerate SVM-based AdaBoost	Machine learning	SVM + AdaBoost	ADNI	95.82% accuracy

6.3 CONCLUSION

Direct strategies for discovering Alzheimer's disease using brain MRI are too expensive and time-consuming. As a result, we extract features and diagnose problems using their categorization and evaluation. This chapter discusses various MR image classification methods in detail including KNN, naive Bayes, SVM, DT, RF, LR, multi-MLP, AdaBoost, and gradient boosting. By reviewing all of the classification methods that are satisfactory in terms of both performance and computational bandwidth and have positive performance for necessary feature separation and object recognition, we can identify the required classifiers. However, as per the review so conducted, it has been observed that there are multiple methods that currently exist in order to detect Alzheimer's disease. Few methods include the implementation of SVM combined with the concepts of DTs, giving an accuracy of 83%. On the other hand, SVM when combined with the fundamentals of ensemble learning such as AdaBoost gives an overall accuracy of detection as 95.82%. However, the parameters used for carrying out the experiment and concluding the accuracy include fine-tuning of algorithms, recall factor, ROC, and AUC curves. Thus, using MRI analysis, traditional classification methods will provide outputs as expected of Alzheimer's patients. This study contributes significantly to the field of brain MRI automatic classification by employing various instantaneous classification techniques. A system like this has the potential to help radiologists and researchers identify AD classification with greater accuracy.

KEYWORDS

- **Alzheimer's disease**
- **machine learning**
- **KNN**
- **random forest**
- **SVM**
- **XGBoost**

REFERENCES

1. Alzheimer's Association. *Alzheimer's and Dementia Diagnosis*; Alzheimer's Association. https://www.alz.org/alzheimersdementia/diagnosis (accessed 15-07-2021).
2. World Health Organization. Dementia. https://www.who.int/news-room/factsheets/detail/dementia (accessed 20-07-2021).
3. Chitradevi, B.; Srimathi, P. An Overview on Image Processing Techniques. *Int. J. Innov. Res. Comput. Commun. Eng.* **2014,** *2*, 6466–6472.
4. Rekhil, M.; Kumar, S. K. A Survey on Image Feature Descriptors. *Int. J. Comput. Sci. Inf. Technol.* **2014,** *5*, 7668–7673.
5. Rabeh, A. B.; Benzarti, F.; Amiri, H. Diagnosis of Alzheimer Diseases in Early Step Using SVM (Support Vector Machine). In *13th International Conference Computer Graphics—Imaging and Visualization*, 2016. DOI: 10.1109/CGiV.2016.76.
6. Asemani, D.; Morsheddost, H.; Shalchy, M. A. Effects of Ageing and Alzheimer Disease on Haemodynamic Response Function: A Challenge for Event-Related fMRI. *Healthc. Technol. Lett.* **2017,** *4* (3), 109–114. DOI: 10.1049/htl.2017.0005.
7. Liu, J.; Wang, J.; Hu, B.; Wu, F.-X.; Pan, Y. Alzheimer's Disease Classification Based on Individual Hierarchical Networks Constructed with 3-D Texture Features. *IEEE Trans. Nanobiosci.* **2017,** *16* (6), 428–437. DOI: 10.1109/TNB.2017.2707139.
8. Zhang, J.; Liu, M.; Le An, Y.G.; Gao, Y.; Shen, D. Alzheimer's Disease Diagnosis Using Landmark-based Features from Longitudinal Structural MR Images. *IEEE J. Biomed. Health Inform.* **2017,** *21* (6), 1607–1616. DOI: 10.1109/JBHI.2017.2704614.
9. Lahmiri, S.; Boukadoum, M. New Approach for Automatic Classification of Alzheimer's Disease, Mild Cognitive Impairment and Healthy Brain Magnetic Resonance Images. *Healthc. Technol. Lett.* **2014,** *1* (1), 32–36. DOI: 10.1049/htl.2013.0022.
10. Reynolds, D. Gaussian Mixture Models. In *Encyclopedia of Biometrics*; Li, S. Z., Jain, A. K., Eds.; Springer: Boston, MA. https://doi.org/10.1007/978-1-4899-7488-4_196
11. Bui, D. T.; Hoang, N. D. A Bayesian Framework Based on a Gaussian Mixture Model and Radial-Basis-Function Fisher Discriminant Analysis. *Geosci. Model Dev.* **2017,** *10* (9), 3391 (BayGmmKda, V., 1) for spatial prediction of floods.
12. Armananzas, R.; Iglesias, M.; Morales, D. A.; Alonso-Nanclares, L. Voxelbased Diagnosis of Alzheimer's Disease Using Classifier Ensembles. *IEEE J. Biomed. Health Inform.* **2017,** *21* (3), 778–784. DOI: 10.1109/JBHI.2016.2538559.
13. Zhu, X.; Sobhani, F.; Xu, C.; Pan, L.; Ghasebeh, M. A.; Kamel, I. R. Quantitative Volumetric Functional MR Imaging: An Imaging Biomarker of Early Treatment Response in Hypo-Vascular Liver Metastasis Patients After Yttrium-90 Transarterial Radioembolization. *Abdom. Radiol. (NY)* **2016,** *41* (8), 1495–1504. DOI: 10.1007/s00261-016-0694-y.
14. Kurth, F.; Gaser, C.; Luders, E. A 12-Step User Guide for Analyzing Voxelwise Gray Matter Asymmetries in Statistical Parametric Mapping (SPM). *Nat. Protoc.* **2015,** *10* (2), 293–304. DOI: 10.1038/nprot.2015.014.
15. Lahmiri, S.; Boukadoum, M. New Approach for Automatic Classification of Alzheimer's Disease, Mild Cognitive Impairment and Healthy Brain Magnetic Resonance Images. *Healthc. Technol. Lett.* **2014,** *1* (1), 32–36. DOI: 10.1049/htl.2013.0022.
16. Srinivasan, A.; Battacharjee, P.; Prasad, A.; Sanyal, G.; Brain, M. R. Image Analysis Using Discrete Wavelet Transform with Fractal Feature Analysis. *IEEE Second*

Int. Conference on Electron., Communication and Aerospace Technology; 2018; pp 1660–1664.
17. Zheng, X.; Shi, J.; Zhang, Q.; Ying, S.; Li, Y. *Improving MRI-Based Diagnosis of Alzheimer's Disease via an Ensemble Privileged Information Learning Algorithm*; IEEE: Ney York, NY; pp 456–459. DOI: 10.1109/ISBI.2017.7950559.
18. Rabeh, A. B.; Benzarti, F.; Amiri, H. Diagnosis of Alzheimer Diseases in Early Step Using SVM (Support Vector Machine). In *13th International Conference Computer Graphics, Imaging and Visualization*, 2016. DOI: 10.1109/CGiV.2016.76.
19. Burbidge, R.; Trotter, M.; Buxton, B.; Holden, S. Drug Design by Machine Learning: Support Vector Machines for Pharmaceutical Data Analysis. *Comput. Chem.* **2001,** 26 (1), 5–14. DOI: 10.1016/s0097-8485(01)00094-8.
20. Valentini, G. Gene Expression Data Analysis of Human Lymphoma Using Support Vector Machines and Output Coding Ensembles. *Artif. Intell. Med.* **2002,** 26 (3), 281–304. DOI: 10.1016/s0933-3657(02)00077-5.
21. L, Shutao, J. T.; Kwok, H.; Zhua, Y.; Wang. Texture Classification Using the Support Vector Machines. *Pattern Recognit.* **2003,** 2883–2893.
22. Saputra, R. A.; Agustina, C.; et al. Detecting Alzheimer's Disease by the Decision Tree Methods Based on Particle Swarm Optimization. *J. Phys. Conf. Ser.* **2020,** *6596*, 1742.
23. Bi, X. A.; Shu, Q.; Sun, Q.; Xu, Q. Random Support Vector Machine Cluster Analysis of Resting-State fMRI in Alzheimer's Disease. *PLoS One* **2018,** *13* (3), e0194479. DOI: 10.1371/journal.pone.0194479.
24. Joshi, S.; Simha, V.; Shenoy, D.; Venugopal, K. R.; Patnaik, L. M. Classification and Treatment of Different Stages of Alzheimer's Disease Using Various Machine Learning Methods. *Int. J. Bioinf. Res.* **2010,** *2* (1), 44–52.
25. Plant, C.; Teipel, S. J.; Oswald, A.; Böhm, C.; Meindl, T.; Mourao-Miranda, J.; Bokde, A. W.; Hampel, H.; Ewers, M. Automated Detection of Brain Atrophy Patterns Based on MRI for the Prediction of Alzheimer's Disease. *Neuroimage* **2010,** *50* (1), 162–174. DOI: 10.1016/j.neuroimage.2009.11.046.
26. Piers, J.; Luke, V.; et al. Genetic Algorithm with Logistic Regression for Prediction of Progression to Alzheimer's Disease. *BMC Bioinf.* **2014,** *15* (Suppl. 11), 1–14. DOI: 10.1186/1471-2105-15-S16-S11.
27. Maggipinto, T.; Bellotti, R.; Amoroso, N.; Diacono, D.; Donvito, G.; Lella, E.; Monaco, A.; Scelsi, M. A.; Tangaro, S. Initiative, A.D.N. DTI Measurements for Alzheimer's Classification. *Phys. Boil.* **2017,** 2361–2375.
28. Sarica, A.; Cerasa, A.; Quattrone, A. Random Forest Algorithm for the Classification of Neuroimaging Data in Alzheimer's Disease: A Systematic Review. *Front. Aging Neurosci.* **2017,** *9*, 329. DOI: 10.3389/fnagi.2017.00329.
29. Dimitriadis, S. I.; Liparas, D.; Tsolaki, M. N.; Alzheimer's Disease Neuroimaging Initiative. Random Forest Feature Selection, Fusion and Ensemble Strategy: Combining Multiple Morphological MRI Measures to Discriminate among Healthy Elderly, MCI, cMCI and Alzheimer's Disease Patients: From the Alzheimer's Disease Neuroimaging Initiative (ADNI) Database. *J. Neurosci. Methods* **2018,** *302*, 14–23. DOI: 10.1016/j.jneumeth.2017.12.010.
30. Rathore, S.; Habes, M.; Iftikhar, M. A.; Shacklett, A.; Davatzikos, C. A Review on Neuroimaging-Based Classification Studies and Associated Feature Extraction

Methods for Alzheimer's Disease and Its Prodromal Stages. *Neuroimage* **2017,** 155, 530–548. DOI: 10.1016/j.neuroimage.2017.03.057.
31. Arbabshirani, M. R.; Plis, S.; Sui, J.; Calhoun, V. D. Single Subject Prediction of Brain Disorders in Neuroimaging: Promises and Pitfalls. *Neuroimage* **2017,** *145* (B), 137–165. DOI: 10.1016/j.neuroimage.2016.02.079.
32. Falahati, F.; Westman, E.; Simmons, A. Multivariate Data Analysis and Machine Learning in Alzheimer's Disease with a Focus on Structural Magnetic Resonance Imaging. *J. Alzheimers Dis.* **2014,** *41* (3), 685–708. DOI: 10.3233/JAD-131928.
33. Dinu, A.; J.; Ganesan, R. Early Detection of Alzheimer's Disease Using Predictive *k*-NN Instance Based Approach and T-Test Method. *Int. J. Adv. Trends Comput. Sci. Eng.* **2019,** *8*, 1.4.
34. Horn, J. F.; Habert, M. O.; Kas, A.; Malek, Z.; Maksud, P.; Lacomblez, L.; Giron, A.; Fertil, B. F. Differential Automatic Diagnosis Between Alzheimer's Disease and Frontotemporal Dementia-Based on Perfusion SPECT Images. *Artif. Intell. Med.* **2009,** *47* (2), 147–158. DOI: 10.1016/j.artmed.2009.05.001.
35. L, Huang, Z.; Pan, H.; Lu. Automated Diagnosis of Alzheimer's Disease with Degenerate SVM-Based AdaBoost. In *5th International Conference on Intelligent Human-Machine Systems and Cybernetics*; 2013; pp 298–301.
36. Carnero-Pardo, C.; Espejo-Martínez, B.; López-Alcalde, S.; Espinosa-García, M.; Sáez-Zea, C.; Hernández-Torres, E.; Navarro-Espigares, J. L.; Vílchez-Carrillo, R. Diagnostic Accuracy, Effectiveness and Cost for Cognitive Impairment and Dementia Screening of Three Short Cognitive Tests Applicable Toilliterates. *PLoS One* **2011,** *6* (11), e27069. DOI: 10.1371/journal.pone.0027069.
37. Williams, J. A.; Weakley, A.; Cook, D. J.; Schmitter-Edgecombe, M. Machine Learning Techniques for Diagnostic Differentiation of Mild Cognitive Impairment and Dementia. In *Advancement of Artificial Intelligence Conference in Expanding the Boundaries of Health Informatics Using Artificial Intelligence*; 2013; pp 71–76.
38. Schmitter-Edgecombe, M.; Parsey, C.; Cook, D. J. Cognitive Correlates of Functional Performance in Older Adults: Comparison of Self-Report, Direct Observation and Performance Based Measures. *J. Int. Neuropsychol. Soc.* **2011,** *17* (5), 853–864. DOI: 10.1017/S1355617711000865.

CHAPTER 7

A New Strategy for the Prediction of Diabetic Retinopathy Using Deep Learning Methods and Firebase Technology

ABDELWAHEB JEBNOUNI[1], AMIRA HADJ FREDJ[1], and JIHENE MALEK[2]

[1]*Electronics and Micro-electronics, University of Monastir, Faculty of Sciences, Monastir, Tunisia*

[2]*Higher Institute of Applied Sciences and Technology, Sousse, Tunisia*

ABSTRACT

Diabetic retinopathy (DR) is diabetes's most intimidating complication that causes permanent blindness if not tackled swiftly. Its early prediction represents a fundamental challenge nowadays, which is crucial for early treatment and prevention success. The DR detection steps need to be simplified to help people prevent from blindness. Unluckily, expert human interpretation is required for the prevention and identification of the DR degree. However, in many adjacent fields, the deep neural network (DNN) approach is applied in a successful way. Utilizing the firebase technology for accumulating a big labeled dataset is capable of reducing the high costs of our application. One of the challenges is to design a platform for increasing, in particular, the accuracy of the DR prevention. A new strategy for DR prediction is to put forward in this chapter through the investigation of DNN methods for classifying the detected DR fundus.

Applied Intelligence for Medical Image Analysis. Aarti, Raju Pal, Mukesh Saraswat, & Himanshu Mittal (Eds.)

After that, it is saved into a firebase station for database size extension. The learning stages will be repeated by our system, based on those results, to raise accuracy and prevent doctors from wrong decisions. Through the use of this methodology, the model achieves 97.3% accuracy for five classes utilizing for Kaggle cloud a standard model.

7.1 INTRODUCTION

Diabetes is a chronic, noncommunicable, and highly prevalent illness which presents significant public health challenges amongst a lot of people around the world.[1] Diabetic patients who are 18–75 years old may have complete loss of vision due to hysterical diabetes. Such a disease type is called DR.[2] As a matter of fact, the World Health Organization has conducted massive research in this area. Their statistics show that in Europe and the USA, 15–17% of total blindness is caused by diabetic retinopathy (DR), even though there is a clear ethnic variation in vision loss. Furthermore, it appears that, broadly, the blindness burden caused by diabetes is remarkably compelling.[3]

As a matter of fact, the retina has a spheric structure, which is made up of subtle layers. These layers are found in the human-eye backside. The retina is located aside a dark circular part, which is known as the macula, and an optic nerve. Basically, the retina processes the visual information through the transmission of the light to neural signals and through the coordination with the brain.[2] The DR can be the result of retina blood vessel injury or retinal microvascular changes which have an effect on the retinal blood vessels. The DR may appear after a long time of diabetes. People with diabetes for more than 20 years are at risk of being affected by 80% compared to healthier people. The DR influences mostly workers, presenting a principal cause of blindness.[4] Consequently, DR's early detection and clinical diagnosis through health check-ups and systematic treatment are vital always to prevent the DR. Providing the appropriate treatment and regular screening will significantly decrease blindness caused by DR to nearly 90%. In 2003, DR was divided by the International Clinical Disease into five severity categories[5]: no apparent retinopathy, mild nonproliferative DR, moderate NPDR, severe NPDR, and proliferative DR (PDR). Healthy fundus images that do not show any DR symptoms are classified as the first level in DR severity grading. On the other hand, the different three successive levels, which differentiated with the PDR grate by few micro aneurysms and intraregional hemorrhages, may proceed quickly to the latest degree that will most probably cause blindness.

Besides, as the authors indicated, the software does not identify other major eye diseases, for example, signs of glaucoma or age-related macular degeneration. Most DR screening programs currently in development using human assessment include these requirements. It is accordingly difficult to appreciate how modern software can safely "replace" human graders in the current DR screening programs at this time.

According to individual risk factors, high-precision training, as well as solid generation, significant research effort has freshly been based upon developing the DR. To learn more complex patterns, and in order to achieve exceptional prediction accuracy, prediagnosis models are applied for various populations and have significant performance for DR prediction using deep neural network (DNN) and machine learning systems via many layers. In particular, DNNs have given an excellent account in advancing the accuracy of classification compared to conventional models.

Our contribution includes

1) supporting medical practitioners for the detection of DR at early disease stages.
2) improving the performance of traditional DNN models through the use of the hyperparameter optimization technique.
3) including the firebase technology to perform DR detection and classification stages.

The rest of our work is as follows. We discuss in Section 7.2 the related work as regards retinopathy prediction, along with related DNN performance. Section 7.3 illustrates our proposed DR prediction model. Later, Section 7.4 discusses some practical issues for the developed model. And finally, in Section 7.5, we summarize and conclude our work. We study the barriers of this work and future research perspectives.

7.2 RELATED WORK

Nowadays, research focuses intensely on checking the quantification of DR and precisely detecting its characteristics like blood vessels and exudates on fundus images. A computer-based algorithm for detecting individual features of fundus images is realized. Image processing methods are widely used in all these works, such as image threshold systems, 2D matched filters, segmentation, and image preprocessing. These systems cannot mix all diabetic-retinopathy characteristics in one entity for the automatic detection and classification of the different stages of normal subjects. The computer-based microaneurysm recognition algorithm is evolved.[6] However, the literature does not expect to identify the DR stage automatically, and a large number of databases are required. An automatic system for detecting abnormal symptoms is proposed in Dandapat et al.[7] The global threshold and the local threshold are applied to segment the exudate lesions from red images. In fact, such methods cannot increase the automatic detection method's function because the fixed permanent point is complicated. The system introduced in Babiuch et al.[8] can only detect and quantify microaneurysms, which can only help detect mild stages.

Concerning the estimation of prediction uncertainty, the initial work as regards the model of DR detection was introduced in Alfian et al.,[9] in which the Bayesian result was utilized to quantify uncertainty in the binary classification of DR. An extra method was proposed in Perais et al.,[10] in which the arbitrary batch normalization was adopted for calculating the model prediction uncertainty for level interval estimation of the DR. As introduced by the authors in Galdran et al.,[11] they used a dataset with multiple labels for each patient, which was produced by various specialists. The dataset can estimate uncertainty to predict professional disagreements in patient diagnosis.

Firebase technology was used for many medical applications. In Mukhopadhyay et al.,[12] file transfer from sender to doctor is done with a compressed Android app. When the size is more extensive, they use a specific algorithm to process the image. The file has been uploaded to firebase, and the sender gets the server from the application. Then, the application receives the list of users registered with it. The same server then allows selecting recipients from its list of users provided. From the perspective of the receiver, the user has a login to the app and can access files or download. Roisudin et al.[13] develop a framework based on firebase to collect data using an android application.

7.3 METHODOLOGY

Deep learning (DL) is actually a prominent machine learning approaches that imitates human knowledge and behavior to provoke adequate information in different scenarios. For instance, DL allows computer models to achieve high classification accuracy in the image processing field, outperforming human performance levels. These models are trained using labeled datasets that will be fed into the neural network layers—starting from the input layer and propagating through the hidden layers. Every neuron in the hidden layer basically uses one nonlinear activation function, which highlights the valuable information only.

The lack of a robust and highly efficient methodology for DR identification in its primary state raises the need for a more rigorous and flexible technique to achieve this goal. Furthermore, exudates are considered as one of the basic steps. Hence, featuring its diagnosis is crucial for rapid DR detection.

Our proposed model of exudate classification includes four fundamental steps as illustrated in Figure 7.1:

- Training datasets and create a model for classification.
- Test the incoming fundus, image.
- Classify this, image.
- Resave the classified image into the firebase.

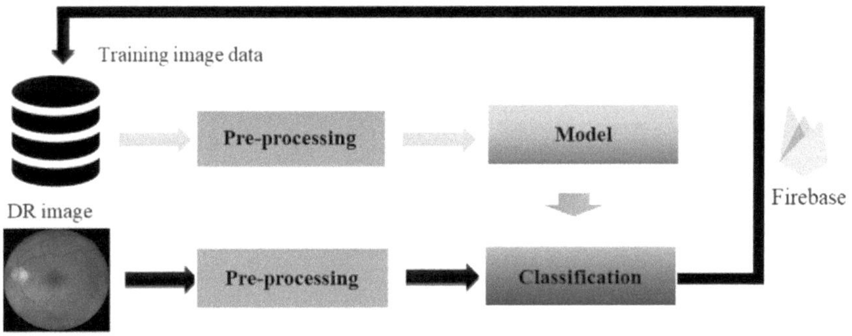

FIGURE 7.1 Block diagram of proposed technique.

7.3.1 DESCRIPTION OF DATASETS

We propose a dataset collected by Kaggle[1] and contains over 80,000 images. The synthesized dataset contains a diverse set of retina images

[1] https://www.kaggle.com/c/diabetic-retinopathy-detection/data

with high resolution, which are obtained through a variety of imaging conditions. As demonstrated in Figure 7.2, the left and right fields are given for each subject. Also, the images are labeled with a subject ID, left or right. For example, the patient ID 1's left eye is 1_left.jpeg. In every image, clinician can rate on a scale of 0–4 in the presence of DR as follows: no DR, mild, moderate, severe, and PDR.

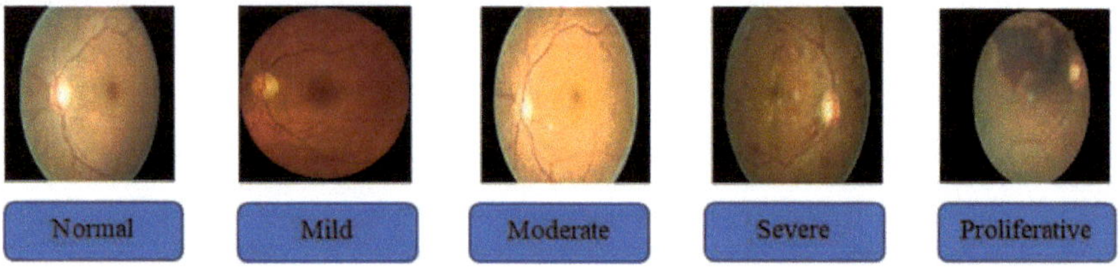

FIGURE 7.2 Fundus photography at each DR severity level: normal, mild, moderate, severe, and proliferative.

The images in the dataset are in fact taken from various models and kinds of cameras (see Table 7.1), which can influence visual left-versus-right representations.

TABLE 7.1 Various Datasets.

Dataset	Images	Resolution	Format	Tasks
Images level annotation[14]	1200	1440 × 960	Images: TIFF diagnosis: excel file	DR grading
Pixel level annotation e-ophtha[15]	148 MAs	2544 × 1696	Images: JPEG	MA small HM detection
Review[16]	1630 normal 46 glaucomatous 16	–	–	Extraction of vessels
DRIONS-DB[17]	110	600 × 400	Images: JPEG	OD
SEED-DB[18]	192 normal 43 glaucomatous	3504 × 2336	–	OD

On the one hand, some of the pictures are presented as seen through the microscope condensing lens (that is to say, inverted as it can be seen in a live eye exam). On the other hand, some images were removed from the dataset if the optic disk is undetectable and the classification is imbalanced due to the image's diversity in each label during the training process. Furthermore, the resolution of retina images in the dataset changes since different fundus cameras took them.

Like any real-world dataset, it encounters unbalanced data and noise in both images and labels. For instance, blurry, underexposed, or overexposed artifacts may be included in these images. This competition aims to generate robust algorithms which could operate successfully despite noise and variation. In Figure 7.3, we present the different class output of data collected by Kaggle for the DR images. It is clear that the first class is the highest class than the other.

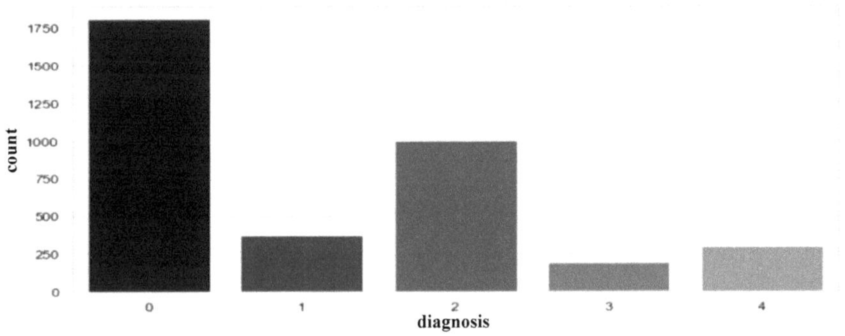

FIGURE 7.3 Class distribution.

7.3.2 PREPROCESSING

Figure 7.4 illustrates the data preparation (data preprocessing) taken into consideration before injecting it into the model. Those steps in the study were retained minimal to prepare a more useful generalization of the image conditions. During the first preprocessing step, we resize every input image into 786 × 512, and we simultaneously keep the aspect ratio with the aim of reducing the training overhead of DNNs using "ImageDataGenerator," a built-in preprocessing function in Keras. It performs a random zoom of 0.15, horizontal/and vertical flip for all the images within the dataset. The image having 512 × 512 size is randomly cropped since it is needed to avoid useless data after resizing the image. In the resultant distributions, each image is clarified using a Gaussian filter before extraction and identification features.

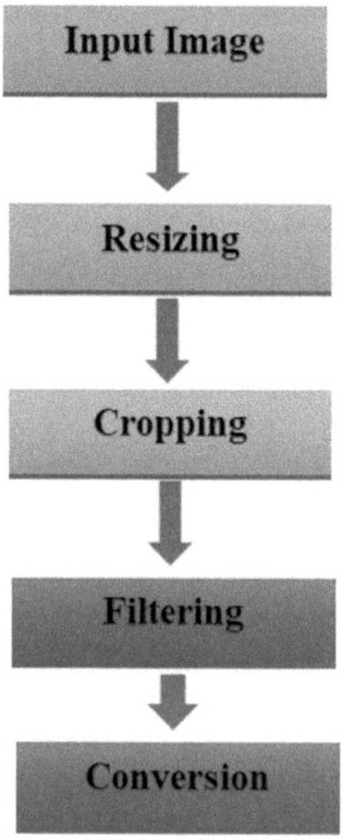

FIGURE 7.4 Different preprocessing steps.

7.3.2.1 GAUSSIAN FILTER

Figure 7.5 illustrates a Gaussian filter which is in fact a 2D convolution operator to be utilized for smoothing images and removing noise.[19]

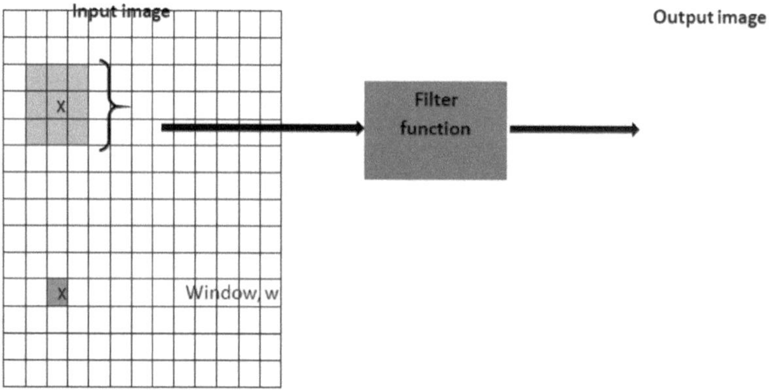

FIGURE 7.5 A window filter. The input window is represented by shaded pixels which deliver the filtered value for a similar location in the output image. Every window position will produce in the output image a similar pixel value.

The convolution of an image $w(x,y)$ of size $m \times n$ with an $f(x,y)$ function designated by $w(x,y) * f(x,y)$ is provided by (7.1)

$$w(x,y)\times f(x,y)=\sum_{s=-a}^{a}\sum_{t=-b}^{-b} w(s,t)\times f(x-s,y-t) \quad (7.1)$$

where a and b are given by: $a=\frac{m-1}{2}$, $b=\frac{n-1}{2}$. Figure 7.4 illustrates a graphical representation of Eq. (7.1). The Gaussian filter is defined by function $f(x,y)$, which is recognized by the Gaussian distribution in the following equation:

$$f(x,y)=\frac{1}{2\pi\sigma}e^{-\frac{x^2-y^2}{2\sigma^2}} \quad (7.2)$$

The Gaussian filter is composed of two parameters: standard deviation σ and window dimensions. The image smoothing effect is higher if the μ value of σ is large. The result of the Gaussian filter is depicted in Figure 7.6.

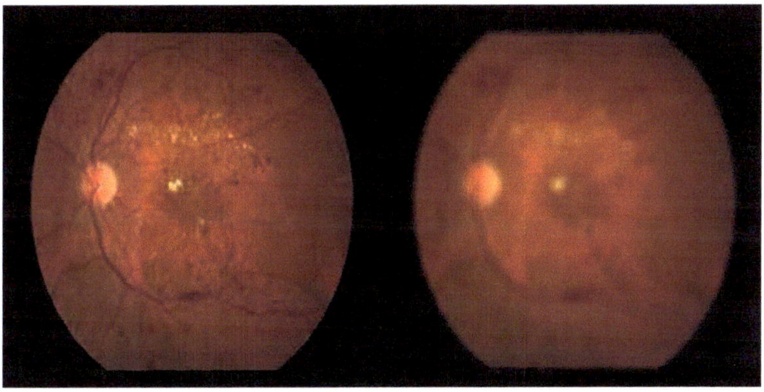

(a) (b)

FIGURE 7.6 (a) Input image and (b) filtered image.

7.3.2.2 RGB TO GRAY

The resulted image is converted to gray scale using the following equation:

$$\text{gray} = 0.3\times \text{R} + 0.59\times \text{G} + 0.11\times \text{B} \quad (7.3)$$

A gray-scale image is just an image in which the exclusive color is gray as shown in Figure 7.7. The idea for dividing this image from any other color image is that more limited data need to be stored for every pixel. Indeed, the "gray" color indicates that the red, green, and blue components all contain a similar intensity in the RGB space, so you just simply need to specify, instead of three intensities, one intensity value for every pixel,[20] and thus specifying every pixel in the full-color image.

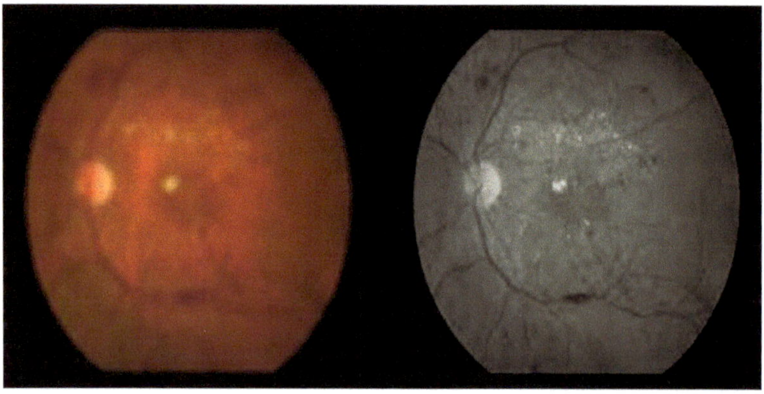

(a) (b)

FIGURE 7.7 (a) RGB image and (b) gray image.

7.4 DATA PROCESSING

7.4.1 DATASET

The synthesized dataset was partitioned into twofolds.[21] The firstfold contains 90% of the dataset, which will be used for training later. What remains is used for validation. The model parameters were adjusted and optimized according to the problem complexity and needs. A separate set of images were used to check the model performance. High-grade classification accuracy was obtained by the method when used to classify the images. Table 7.2 presents the various classes.

TABLE 7.2 Dataset: Distribution of Different Classes

Class	No DR	Mild	Moderate	Severe	PDR	Total
Total	25,810	2443	5292	873	708	35,126
Training	23,229	2199	4753	87	638	30,906
Validation	2580	244	539	786	70	4220

7.4.2 MODEL TRAINING

The functional description profoundly affects the performance of any machine learning model, and the corresponding description applies to the model used for DR identification. With this inspiration, we proposed the model presented in Figure 7.8 to extract the best features from a given retinal image.

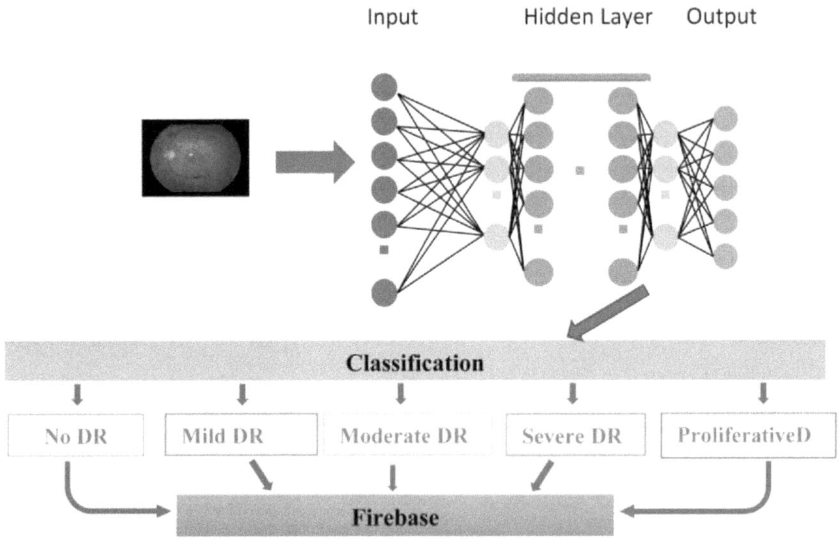

FIGURE 7.8 Block diagram of proposed model.

7.4.2.1 FEATURE EXTRACTION

In this stage, feature extraction aims to convert ready data into a low-dimensional characteristic.[22] According to the label information level, feature extraction can be described as unsupervised, supervised, and semi-supervised feature extraction. This step is carried out to reduce all unnecessary information and to decrease the dimensionality of the feature vector.

In this work, we use this network and provide an image to further propagate to the last max-pooling layer (before the fully connected layers), including selecting the activations at that layer (see Table 7.3).

For the DR severity classification process, we train the model with in-depth blended pretrained features using DNN that contains three hidden layers with 253, 253, and 128 ReLU units, respectively. For the input layer, we applied 0.2 dropout to prevent the model from overfitting, improving model prediction and accuracy.

TABLE 7.3 Model Summary.

Layer (type)	Output shape	Param Number
conv2d (Conv2D)	(None, 255, 255, 32)	896
conv2d_1 (Conv2D)	(None, 253, 253, 32)	9248
max_pooling2d (MaxPooling2D)	(None, 126, 126, 32)	0
dropout (Dropout)	(None, 126, 126, 32)	0
conv2d_2 (Conv2D)	(None, 126, 126, 64)	18496
conv2d_3 (Conv2D)	(None, 124, 124, 64)	36928
max_pooling2d_1 (MaxPooling2)	(None, 62, 62, 64)	0
dropout_1 (Dropout)	(None, 62, 62, 64)	0
conv2d_4 (Conv2D)	(None, 62, 62, 64)	36928
conv2d_5 (Conv2D)	(None, 60, 60, 64)	36928
max_pooling2d_2 (MaxPooling2)	(None, 30, 30, 64)	0
dropout_2 (Dropout)	(None, 30, 30, 64)	0
flatten (Flatten)	(None, 57600)	0
dense (Dense)	(None, 512)	29491712
dropout_3 (Dropout)	(None, 512)	0
dense_1 (Dense)	(None, 5)	2565

7.4.2.2 CLASSIFICATION

To predict diseases like DR, decision-making is performed through the use of decision tree-based approaches.[23] In general, the goal is to create one model that predicts in a correct way the value of target variables. This is done by learning decision rules that are actually inferred from the data features. Our classification can be served by identifying the hyperplane, which facilitates precisely classifying five classes of data points. We compress the linear function output into a vector of five variables, using the sigmoid function. In view of the fact, each compressed value will be more significant than a 0.5 threshold value. After that, we assign a label of 1. Else, the threshold value will be 0. If the linear function output is greater than 1, we will then identify and classify it to belong to a particular class. However, when a result is −1, it will be taken into account as part of another class.

7.5 RESULTS AND PERFORMANCE ANALYSIS

In this research work, a personal computer having 16 GB RAM and Nvidia 1660 Ti with 6 GB was adopted for conducting the experimentation using Python. The network was trained with GPU support training. Our model can function normally with dense feature images. In this suggested DNN structure, compared with every feature detector, each convolutional layer in all three sets that have 64 characteristic detectors is a convolution feature map.

7.5.1 RESULT

A final feature map comes after the hidden layer convolution is unrolled into a single vector with five variables. Each variable is corresponding to the DR level from no DR class to proliferative class. Figures 7.9–7.14 present the prediction of each fundus image.

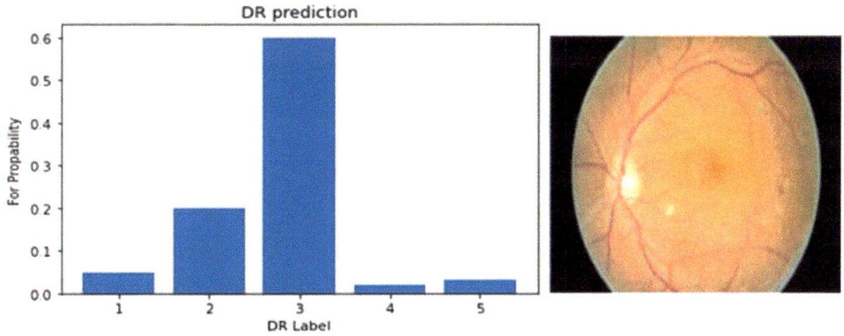

FIGURE 7.9 Classification of normal DR.

7.5.2 METRICS FOR EVALUATION OF THE MODEL

In our classification performance, to prove the developed system efficiency, four metrics are used: accuracy, precision, recall, and specificity. These metrics can be as follows:

$$\text{Accuracy} = (\text{TPR} + \text{TNR}) / (\text{TPR} + \text{TNR} + \text{FPR} + \text{FNR})$$
$$\text{Precision} = \text{TPR} / (\text{TPR} + \text{FPR})$$
$$\text{Recall} = \text{TPR} / (\text{TPR} + \text{FNR})$$
$$\text{Specificity} = \text{TNR} / (\text{FNR} + \text{TNR})$$

where TPR (true positive rate) defines the DR class which is correctly detected, FPR (false positive rate) makes up, in particular, detected objects that do not represent the expected class, and FNR (false negative rate) describes the wrong class. Those metrics are utilized for measuring the detection phase performance for different DR classes that are exposed in Table 7.4.

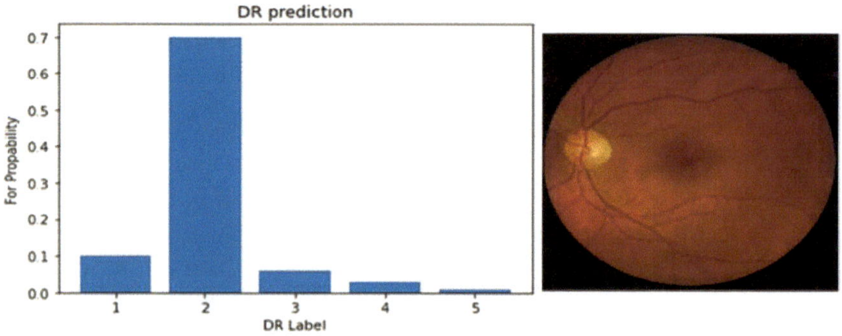

FIGURE 7.10 Classification of mild DR.

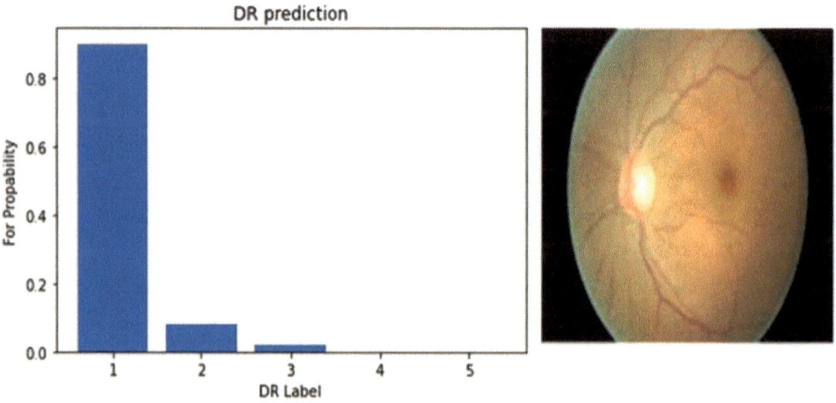

FIGURE 7.11 Classification of moderate DR.

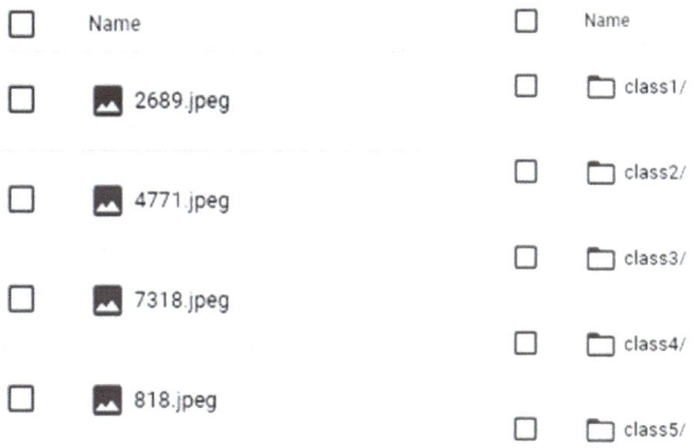

FIGURE 7.12 Classification of severe DR.

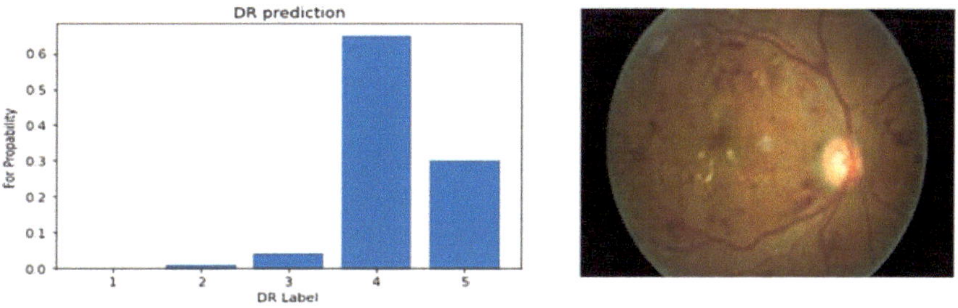

FIGURE 7.13 Classification of proliferative DR.

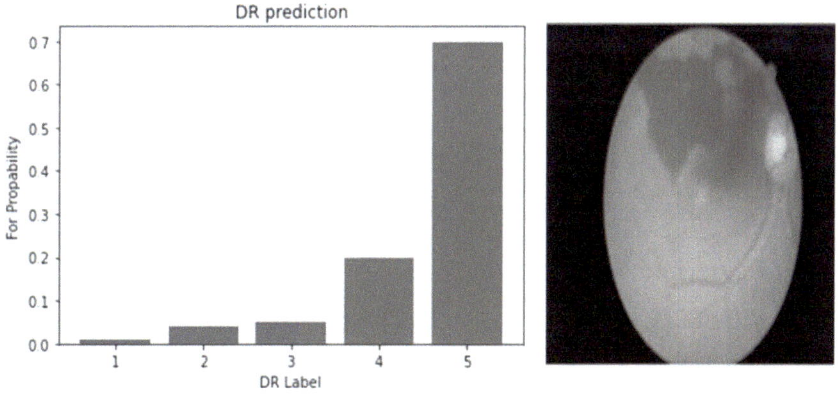

FIGURE 7.14 Result data saved in firebase.

TABLE 7.4 Result Performance.

Accuracy	Precision	Recall	Specificity
94.8%	97.3 %	94.7 %	98%

Comparison classifications from different DNN models are shown in Table 7.5.

TABLE 7.5 Performance between Various DNN Models.

Model	Specificity	Recall	Accuracy
AlexNet	90.07%	79.68%	73.04%
GoogleNet	86.84%	77.56%	82.18%
Resnet	90.53%	82.66%	78.68%
Proposed model	98%	94.7%	94.8%

We evaluate our proposed model with some standard model. According to Table 7.5, we remark that our model has a better accuracy, recall, and specificity rate than the other models.

Table 7.6 presents test evaluation of accuracy metric applied for 100 images for each class. We remark that our model is less than 94% for the normal DR and severe DR classes; however, it is greater than 95% for the moderate and ser DR classes.

TABLE 7.6 Accuracy Metric for DR Classes.

Class	Accuracy
Normal DR	92%
Mild DR	94%
Moderate DR	97%
Severe DR	91%
Proliferative DR	100%

7.6 CONCLUSION

Early detection of DR is helpful to successfully recover from this disease. However, diagnostic processes are expensive and time-consuming to analyze and scrutinize medical images in computers, have a high-speed processing capacity, and can provide better forecast accuracy. In this chapter, we have made up a computational model for predicting DR. For clinical diagnosis, accuracy prediction and several performance measurements are relatively high and reliable. Classifying the performance model mainly depends upon datasets and feature preprocessing extraction methods. This model will be implemented in the future into a hardware platform to perform system predictions.

KEYWORDS

- **deep neural networks**
- **diabetic retinopathy**
- **firebase**
- **fundus**

REFERENCES

1. Preshaw, P. M.; Bissett, S. M. Periodontitis and Diabetes. *B.D.J. Team* **2020,** *7* (5), 27–35.
2. Mateen, M.; Wen, J.; Hassan, M.; Nasrullah, N.; Sun, S.; Hayat, S. Automatic Detection of Diabetic Retinopathy: A Review on Datasets, Methods and Evaluation Metrics. *IEEE Access.* **2020,** *8*, 48784–48811. DOI: 10.1109/ACCESS.2020.2980055.
3. Resnikoff, S.; Pascolini, D.; Mariotti, S. P.; Pokharel, G. P. J. Global Magnitude of Visual Impairment Caused by Uncorrected Refractive Errors in 2004. *Bull. World Health Organ.* **2008,** *86* (1), 63–70. DOI: 10.2471/blt.07.041210.
4. Islam, K. T.; Wijewickrema, S.; O'Leary, S., Eds. Identifying Diabetic Retinopathy from OCT Images Using Deep Transfer Learning with Artificial Neural Networks. In *2019 32nd International Symposium on Computer-Based Medical Systems (CBMS)*; IEEE: New York, NY, 2019. DOI: 10.1109/CBMS.2019.00066.
5. Wilkinson, C. P.; Ferris III, F. L.; Klein, R. E.; Lee, P. P.; Agardh, C. D.; Davis, M.; Dills, D.; Kampik, A.; Pararajasegaram, R.; Verdaguer, J. T.; Global Diabetic Retinopathy Project Group. Proposed International Clinical Diabetic Retinopathy and Diabetic Macular Edema Disease Severity Scales. *Ophthalmology* **2003,** *110* (9), 1677–1682. DOI: 10.1016/S0161-6420(03)00475-5.
6. Antal, B.; Hajdu, A. An Ensemble-Based System for Microaneurysm Detection and Diabetic Retinopathy Grading. *IEEE Trans. Biomed. Eng.* **2012,** *59* (6), 1720–1726. DOI: 10.1109/TBME.2012.2193126.

7. Dandapat, S.; Ghosh, S.; Si, S.; Datta, A., Eds. Analysis of Diabetic Retinopathy Abnormalities Detection Techniques. In *Proceedings of the International Conference on Frontiers in Computing and Systems*; Springer: Cham, 2021; pp 235–247. DOI: 10.1007/978-981-15-7834-2_22.
8. Babiuch, A.; Wykoff, C. C.; Hach, J.; Srivastava, S.; Talcott, K. E.; Hannah, J. Y.; et al. Longitudinal Panretinal Microaneurysm Dynamics on Ultra-Widefield Fluorescein Angiography in Eyes Treated with Intravitreal Aflibercept for Proliferative Diabetic Retinopathy in the Recovery Study. *Br. J. Ophthalmol.* **2021,** *105* (8), 1111–1115.
9. Alfian, G.; Syafrudin, M.; Fitriyani, N. L.; Anshari, M.; Stasa, P.; Svub, J.; et al. Deep Neural Network for Predicting Diabetic Retinopathy from Risk Factors. *Mathematics* **2020,** *8* (9), 1620.
10. Perais, J.; Agarwal, R.; Hogg, R.; Lawrenson, J. G.; Evans, J. R.; Takwoingi, Y.; et al. Prognostic Factors for the Development and Progression of Proliferative Diabetic Retinopathy in People with Diabetic Retinopathy. *Cochrane Database Syst. Rev.* **2020,** *11*. DOI: 10.1002/14651858.CD013775.pub2.
11. Galdran, A.; Dolz, J.; Chakor, H.; Lombaert, H.; Ayed, I. B., Eds. Cost-Sensitive Regularization for Diabetic Retinopathy Grading from Eye Fundus Images. In *International Conference on Medical Image Computing and Computer-Assisted Intervention*; Springer: Cham, 2020.
12. Mukhopadhyay, A.; Shaji, R. P.; Raj, A., Eds. Delay Reduced Multimedia Transmission in Medical Emergencies International Conference on Advances in Computing. In *2018 Communications and Informatics (ICACCI)*; IEEE Publications: New York, 2018; Vol. 2018. DOI: 10.1109/ICACCI.2018.8554907.
13. Nugroho, R. A.; Kartini, A.; Prasetijo, A. B. J. I. JoH, Education, Social. Designing an Android-Based Diabetes Health Reminder Educational. *Inf. Syst.* **2020,** *3* (10), 1–21.
14. Decencière, E.; Zhang, X.; Cazuguel, G.; Lay, B.; Cochener, B.; Trone, C.; Gain, P.; Ordonez, R.; Massin, P.; Erginay, A.; Charton, B.; Klein, J. Feedback on a Publicly Distributed Image Database: The Messidor Database. *Image Anal. Stereol.* **2014,** *33* (3), 231–234. DOI: 10.5566/ias.1155.
15. Decencière, E.; Cazuguel, G.; Zhang, X.; Thibault, G.; Klein, J.-C.; Meyer, F.; Marcotegui, B.; Quellec, G.; Lamard, M.; Danno, R.; Elie, D.; Massin, P.; Viktor, Z.; Erginay, A.; Laÿ, B.; Chabouis, A. TeleOphta: Machine Learning and Image Processing Methods for Teleophthalmology. *IRBM* **2013,** *34* (2), 196–203. DOI: 10.1016/j.irbm.2013.01.010.
16. Habib, M.; Steel, D.; Al-Diri, B.; Hunter, A.; Hudaib, T.; Berry, S., Eds. A Reference Data Set for Retinal Vessel Profiles. In *30th Annual International Conference of the IEEE Engineering in Medicine and Biology Society (EMBS)*; Newcastle University: Newcastle, 2008.
17. Sivaswamy, J.; Krishnadas, S. R.; Datt Joshi, G.; Jain, M.; Syed Tabish, A. U., Eds. Drishti-gs: Retinal Image Dataset for Optic Nerve Head (ONH) Segmentation. In *2014 11th International Symposium on Biomedical Imaging (ISBI)*; IEEE: New York, NY, 2014. DOI: 10.1109/ISBI.2014.6867807.
18. Park, R.; Roman, L.; Falardeau, L.; Albino, L.; Joye, I.; Martinez, M. M. J. F. High Temperature Rotational Rheology of the Seed Flour to Predict the Texture of Canned Red Kidney Beans (*Phaseolus vulgaris*). *Foods* **2020,** *9* (8), 1002. DOI: 10.3390/foods9081002.

19. Haddad, R. A.; Akansu, A. N. A Class of Fast Gaussian Binomial Filters for Speech and Image Processing. *IEEE Trans. Signal Process.* **1991,** *39* (3), 723–727.
20. Li, S.; Li, D.; Zhang, C.; Wan, J.; Xie, M. J. S. RGB-D Image Processing Algorithm for Target Recognition and Pose Estimation of Visual Servo System. *Sensors (Basel)* **2020,** *20* (2), 430. DOI: 10.3390/s20020430.
21. Yu, F.; Xu, Z.; Shen, T.; Stamoulis, D.; Shangguan, L.; Wang, D.; et al. Towards Latency-Aware DNN Optimization with GPU Runtime Analysis and Tail Effect Elimination. *arXiv* **2020**. arXiv:2011.03897.
22. Liu, Z.; Lai, Z.; Ou, W.; Zhang, K.; Zheng, R. J. S. P. Structured Optimal Graph Based Sparse Feature Extraction for Semi-Supervised Learning. *Signal Process.* **2020,** *170*, 107456. DOI: 10.1016/j.sigpro.2020.107456.
23. Cuesta, H. A.; Coffman, D. L.; Branas, C.; Murphy, H. M. Using Decision Trees to Understand the Influence of Individual- and Neighborhood-Level Factors on Urban Diabetes and Asthma. *Health Place* **2019,** *58*, 102119.

CHAPTER 8

Contactless Monitoring in Newborns Using Infrared Thermography: A Review

LALIT MAURYA[1,2], ROOP SINGH[2], DEEPAK CHAWLA[3], and PRASANT MAHAPATRA[1,2]

[1]*Academy of Scientific and Innovative Research (AcSIR), Ghaziabad, Uttar Pradesh, India*

[2]*Biomedical Application (BMA) Group, CSIR-Central Scientific Instruments Organisation (CSIR-CSIO), Chandigarh, Haryana, India*

[3]*Department of Neonatology, Government Medical College & Hospital (GMCH), Chandigarh, Haryana, India*

ABSTRACT

In neonatal care, the monitoring of temperature, heart rate, and breathing rate plays a pivotal role in determining the neonate's health status and medical diagnosis. However, the existing contact-based methods confront challenges such as discomfort, skin infections, and altering sleep patterns. Infrared imaging is very useful in temperature-related physiological changes' measurement with the characteristic of noncontact, nonradiative, and functional method.

This chapter describes and explains infrared thermography (IRT) used in the monitoring of vital physiological parameters of neonatal. Due to its use as portable and reliable, the IRT will be easily implemented for monitoring the neonate's body surface temperature and breathing rate. The chapter indicates IRT as a new era of research in neonate monitoring and has a broad future in medical imaging.

Applied Intelligence for Medical Image Analysis. Aarti, Raju Pal, Mukesh Saraswat, & Himanshu Mittal (Eds.)

8.1 INTRODUCTION

The first four weeks of life is a crucial time for the newborn, is termed neonatal period, and needs extra care.[1] Globally, neonatal mortality is declining during the last four decades. However, the neonatal mortality rate is declining slowly in most low-income countries, including India, and progress toward achieving Millennium Development Goal 4 with the objective of reducing child mortality[2] is on a moderate scale. To speed up progress, it is important that preventing neonatal deaths has been put in order of importance. Neonatal monitoring is the process of monitoring key physiological changes in infants (newborns) born with various conditions, including premature birth, infection, surgical complications, breathing, and heart anomalies. Newborns who face complications due to prematurity or infection may have long-term problems and are also required to be monitored for a long period of time after delivery.

The newborn regulates its own body temperature much less efficiently than adults and therefore easily cools down or heat up much faster—the smaller and more premature the baby, the greater the risk. Keeping up a stable micro-environment is one of the key physiologic difficulties that an infant must face after delivery. Thermal stress in a newborn has been identified as a key cause of increased morbidity and mortality, emphasizing the importance of early diagnosis by thermoregulation monitoring.[3] The World Health Organization has issued a practical guideline for newborn thermal safety. It suggests a variety of linked techniques to promote neonatal thermal preservation, which is called as "warm chain."[4] It is also required that the monitoring system is not only limited to neonatal intensive care unit (NICU) but also portable and suitable for keep monitoring in different interlinked procedures of "warm chain."

Respiratory distress is one of the most common causes for a newborn to be admitted to the NICU and needs continuous monitoring of breath rate and respiratory behaviors.[5] However, respiratory distress monitoring is not limited to premature newborns. It is increasingly common in postneonatal and modest prematurity.

For neonatal monitoring, many contact-based technologies have been suggested.[6–10] Raj et al.[11] suggested a simple, cost-effective technology but encountered an issue with the sensor's adhesion. Contact-based methods introduce a number of complications, including pain, the possibility of skin injury, and infections.[12] Additionally, for premature babies or newborns, there is the risk of skin damage from the detachment of the electrode. It emphasizes the importance of implementing a contactless approach that could be used in clinical settings. Contactless monitoring has attracted increased interest in newborns and appears to be a promising choice for addressing the difficulties associated with traditional contact monitoring.[13] In the noncontact method, the body temperature and breathing rate are measured remotely, without any physical contact with the body. Contactless breathing monitoring systems have evident advantages.[14,15] It improves the patient's comfort (particularly for long-term monitoring of neonates and rehabilitation patients) and reduces the possibility of inaccurate measurement as distress caused by the contact device or adhesive sensor may alter the breathing rate and body temperature measurement. One of the noncontact techniques for breathing rate is Doppler radar.[16] This approach is usually subjected by the radiation, the bulkiness, and the extreme susceptibility to motion artifacts. Recently, the focus is broadened by introducing imaging techniques: visible,[17] remote-photoplethysmography,[18] and thermal imaging.[14]

Every object having a temperature above absolute zero temperature emits electromagnetic waves in the infrared (IR) range called thermal radiation. Infrared thermography (IRT), simply called thermal imaging, records the IR radiation emitted by the body and, by using this radiation profile, visualizes the temperature profile of the body. The thermal camera captures this thermal profile either in white-hot or in different color palettes. Thermal imaging can easily illustrate the variation in body surface temperature, making it useful for the early identification and diagnosis of several diseases. In medical diagnosis, thermal imaging is a noncontact, noninvasive, nonradiative method for analyzing the physiological function related to the thermoregulation of the body or organ temperature. With the advancement of IR sensors, optics, electronics, and software, it has been used in the detection and assessment of various diseases like breast cancer, arthritis, diabetes, wound, and inflamed joints. However, there are still many challenges of thermal imaging in medical diagnostic research and in developing a controlled environment for accurate acquisition.[19] Additionally, integration with other technology is also a challenge for researchers.

In this chapter, the scope of contactless body surface temperature and respiration monitoring using IRT in the newborn is reviewed. Section 8.2 describes the working of IRT, the history, and evolution of the IRT cameras. Section 8.3 reviews the use of IRT in medical diagnosis. Section 8.4 reviews the IRT in newborns. Finally, the scope of this work and future direction is explained in Section 8.5.

8.2 INFRARED THERMOGRAPHY

8.2.1 HISTORICAL PERSPECTIVE

Traditionally, the human measured the body temperature by using thermistors, thermocouples, and thermopiles put on the specific area of the skin. However, these sensors are difficult to attach and are slow to respond. Additionally, it is not possible to simultaneously measure on the adjacent skin surfaces. Also, the sensor contact is susceptible to any form of movement. In contrast, a thermal camera can remotely measure the entire body surface temperature, which is visualized in the two-dimensional plane.

Sir Herschel[20] was the first to discover the wave range beyond the visual range that can be used to quantify temperature or heat profiles. Sir John Herschel, the son of William Herschel, delivered the main temperature or heat illustration in 1840 from sun-oriented radiation.[21] He defined a term for it called "thermogram," which is also used today to illustrate the temperature distribution in an object. In the earlier days, thermograms were not visually pleasing, took a long time to respond, and were only available in black and white. The evolution of thermal cameras has a major role in the improvement of quality in thermal imaging. Earlier research in IRT was mainly focused on the development of sensors with aiming efficiency as a major factor. The application of the thermal imaging was also limited to military and defense purposes. The technology was classified and highly secret during that time period. Lawson documented the first thermal image processing for a cancer patient by observing the temperature difference of cancer spots from other normal parts.[22] Nowadays, researchers and physicians are using thermography to explore a variety of different illness problems, including breast cancer, skin cancer, and thyroid disease.

8.2.2 HOW IRT WORKS

A thermogram or thermal image depicts how much IR radiation an object radiates, transfers, and reflects. Thermal images are used to depict temperature variation because the amount of IR radiation emitted increases as the temperature rises. IR radiation, which is found between visible and microwave, is part of the electromagnetic spectrum. The electromagnetic spectrum is partitioned into different wavelength groups, termed bands, that are recognized by the strategies utilized to create and identify radiation inside each band.

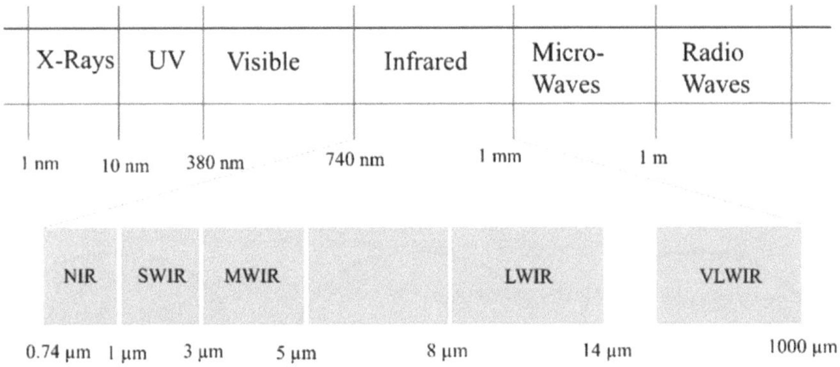

FIGURE 8.1 The visualization of a specified subdivision of infrared range in the electromagnetic (EM) spectrum.

These groups are called X-ray (<10 nm), ultraviolet (<380 nm), visible (<780 nm), IR (<1 mm), microwave (<30 cm), and radio-wave (<10 km, 30 kHz) bands (Fig. 8.1). Further, the IR is classified as near-IR (740 nm–1 μm), short-wave IR (1–3 μm), mid-wave IR (3–5 μm), and long-wave IR (8–12 μm). Thermal imaging measures the IR radiation emitted by a body in the 8–14 μm (LWIR) range and illustrates the temperature profile of that body's surface.[23] The thermal camera or sensor is used to record the thermal profile of the object in the form of an image. The image represents the quantified temperature or radiation value of emitted IR radiation at each spatial position of an object. The radiation energy captured by the thermal camera to determine the temperature is dependent on the body's temperature and emissivity. The ratio of an object's emitted energy to the emitted energy of the black body at an equivalent temperature is defined as the emissivity.

The black body can radiate maximum energy and work as the reference to specify the body. In the wavelength range of 2–14 μm, the emissivity of human skin is about 0.97–0.98.[24] In general, the IR camera has an optical system, one or more sensor mechanisms and detectors to convert captured IR energy into electrical energy, some systems for scanning mechanism (currently, there is no requirement of this), a processor, and a display unit as shown in Figure 8.2. The working of an optical system is the same as a visible camera optical system; however, the material is specific for IR wavelength. The sensor mechanism (thermal detector) is the key element of the thermal camera. Nowadays, the photon or quantum detectors are usually referred, and for details about the technology, one can refer *Handbook of Infrared Detection Technologies*.[25] Some preprocessing is performed by the processor inbuilt in camera to set the thresholding, nonuniformity correction, and pseudocoloring. Typically, the image captured by the thermal camera is viewed on a separate external monitor, which could be a computer screen or a small screen embedded with camera.

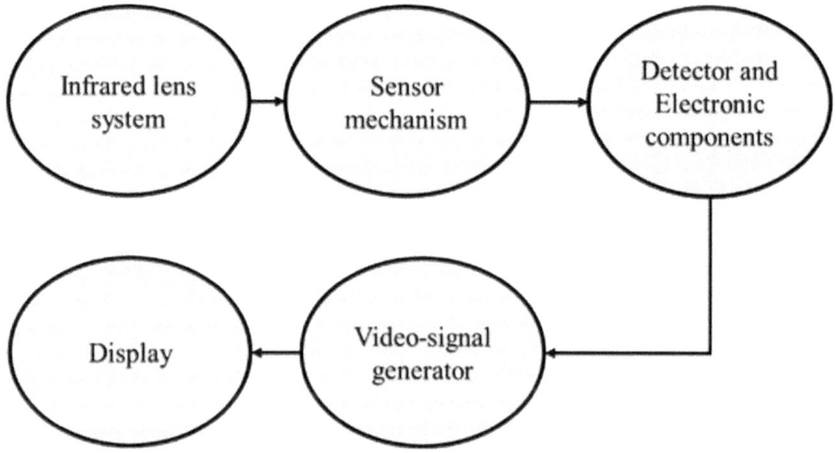

FIGURE 8.2 Overview of the components in thermal camera.[26]

8.2.3 EVOLUTION OF IR CAMERAS

The common purpose of all thermal cameras is to transform IR radiation into visual images.[27] The earliest generation of thermal cameras was big in size and included single element detector. This was improved by utilizing the array of around 120 elements. Later, a camera having detector elements arranged in rows and columns was used to obtain the two-dimensional visualization. The latest generation cameras upgraded the accuracy and performance by utilizing large-size focal plane array and integrating of image computing capabilities.[28,29] These have predominant temperature affectability, speed of operation, and spatial determination than prior adaptations.[27] The first-generation thermal cameras were huge, cooled with liquid nitrogen, requiring liquid nitrogen cooling, and had to be kept horizontal to prevent nitrogen from falling on the subject.[23] Currently, available cameras are smaller, simple to manage, free from orientation, and there is no need of liquid nitrogen because no refrigeration is required. Thermal cameras can produce both videos and digital images of any object. The video records the temperature variation of any object with time.

8.3 IRT IN MEDICAL DIAGNOSIS

Despite the fact that IRT has been used by researchers in the aviation, military, and mechanical industries, it is relatively new in the medical field. The thermal image of the human body illustrates the body's temperature anomaly. Medical diagnosis is based on structural and functional information of the patient, as well as subjective symptoms. In general, structural information is obtained through imaging techniques such as ultrasound, classical microscopy, X-ray, and magnetic resonance imaging. Functional methods are like an electroencephalogram, pulmonary air flow tests, and thermal imaging. IRT is a contactless, noninvasive, and nonradiative technique for measuring the physiological function related to the body's thermal regulation or organ temperature in medical diagnostics.

Clinicians and researchers have recently studied novel and interesting applications with a wide range of clinical consequences, including the study of asymmetric body temperature distributions, which may play a role in the pathophysiology of a variety of diseases.[30–33] Additionally, the distribution of body temperature contributes as a measure of emotions and expression.[34,35] Despite the limited investigation of thermal imaging in the pediatric populace particularly on neonates, numerous of the thermal imaging-based methodologies utilized in grown-ups have potential and may be well suited for newborn children.

The human body's core behaves as a thermal reservoir, and a reasonable temperature remains under normal circumstances. Heat transfers from the bloodstream to the skin through the blood vessels. The rate of heat exchange between the core and the surrounding environment via radiation, conduction, convection, and evaporation regulates the temperature of the skin's surface.[36,37] A normal healthy adult should have symmetrical skin temperature distribution across the body. Thermal IRT may reveal the asymmetry in temperature distribution caused by the perfusion abnormalities.[38–40] Moreover, it is useful in the study of medical conditions related to changes in body temperature induced by vasodilation or constriction, hypothermia or hyperthermia, hypoperfusion or hyperperfusion, and hypermetabolism or hypervascularization.[38,39]

In specific, researchers and doctors have used IRT to detect and evaluate cancerous tumors. Mital et al.[33] developed a technique that uses IRT to assess the depth and location of a breast tumor. Another application of thermal imaging is the detection of fever when mass screening occurs during pandemic-like situations. Clinicians utilized this technology in China during the peak of pandemic for the purpose of mass screening.[41,42] Since thermal cameras are compact, light, and precise, it can rapidly measure the temperature of a large number of people without being exposed to people who are infected by potential infectious diseases.

Researchers have too utilized infrared imaging to analyze thyroid infections,[38] affirm hydrocephalus shunt patency,[43] evaluate the treatment of diabetic wounds,[31] and analyze and diagnose leg ulcers.[32] In sport studies, analysts were utilized IRT to map out temperature disparities during workout and rest.[44]

8.4 IRT IN NEONATES

R. B. Barnes[45] investigated thermal imaging as a new concept for contactless temperature monitoring of the human body using infrared-radiant energy. His research hypothesized that by recording infrared radiation as a thermogram, he might build a precise temperature map of the skin. The skin temperatures were mostly derived by the vascularity of the skin and the heat transferred from within the body if the naked patient kept stationary in a cool environment for 10–15 min prior to thermal imaging. The resulting temperature map provides information on specific pathological states within the body, because the contrasts that develop under these settings are primarily due to internal sources of heat.

Clark and Stothers[46] pioneered the use of IRT on neonates in the year 1980. They used IRT to determine the distribution of neonatal skin temperature. They found that the arms, thighs, and buttocks of newborn have a mean value and are susceptible to changes in ambient temperature. They concluded that the skin that covers the upper abdomen is heated and is generally insensitive to changes in ambient temperature than the mean skin temperature.

Following that, more researchers focused on the scope of thermal imaging on newborns. Anderson et al.[47] investigated the use of thermal imaging to study children who sleep at home. First, the body temperature was recorded, and thermography was performed on five children, four of whom were sleeping in similar conditions for ambient temperature and isolation, and resultant thermography patterns were similar to deep body temperature. The other slept in more hotter conditions and made a diverse thermogenic reaction.[48] They concluded the potential possibilities of thermal imaging to observe the body temperature variations and body movements at home.

Adams et al.[49] developed a novel method for demonstrating the feasibility of using infrared thermographic calorimetry (ITC) to assess the energy expenditure of premature babies, as compared to the respiratory indirect calorimetry. ITC is a measurement of the average surface temperature of the child's body. ITC has been used in conjunction with the heat loss theory to compute radiant heat losses, convection, evaporation, and conduction losses, thus determining the total energy consumption. They concluded that the ITC was an accurate and noninvasive approach for determining heat loss and energy expenditure in healthy premature infants and hence may be used as a clinical and diagnostic tool.

Furthermore, Christidis et al.[50] conducted an interesting study on IRT in neonates during the first hour after childbirth. They measured the surface temperature of a newborn from the time of birth to the first hour. Additionally, the impact of a variety of environmental factors on surface temperature has been demonstrated. Thermal imaging is a simple tool for depicting a person's temperature profile, according to their research. It could be useful to optimize the environmental conditions in delivery rooms and newborn critical care units, without requiring direct contact with the skin. However, thermal imaging revealed the newborn's whole body surface temperature but not the core temperature.

Further, the IRT was used to measure the skin temperature of the newborn on different positions and postures, including kangaroo maternal care.[51] IRT is also a valuable strategy for noncontact physiological monitoring of breathing. By using IRT, it is possible to record the average thermal airflow of the patient's nostrils, related to breathing. The nostrils are recognized and defined as a region of interest (ROI), which is then automatically tracked throughout the measurement procedure employing image processing methods. This technology is a promising option for passive contactless monitoring of respiratory activity in preterm infants and may be used in conjunction with IRT-based newborn temperature monitoring.

In recent years, the researchers investigated the potential, advances, and limitation of thermal imaging for the purpose of breathing monitoring. A study on premature babies for respiration monitoring using IRT measurement has been reported by Abbas et al.[52] They manually selected the nostril region as ROI for respiration rate (RR) detection. A pilot study was performed in Klaessens et al.,[53] in which a simple MATLAB code was used to calculate RR by using infrared imaging. The study's validity was established by the use of an electrocardiogram (ECG)-based technique. This had an excellent agreement in visual results.[53] Another noteworthy technique performed on premature neonates[54] proved reliable. It tracked newborn motion using a particle-filter-based object tracker. A Butterworth filtering was performed for further processing and RR evaluation. The methodology is so easy and feasible and it has a high-level agreement. Likewise, Pereira et al.[5] proposed a technique for newborn infants that used the "Black Box Algorithm" for automatic ROI detection. Since there is no longer anatomical structure to assist in facial recognition, this algorithm works even without a frontal view as compared to the work reported in Abbas et al.[52]

Researchers at Carleton University in Canada performed a study on thermal imaging for the diagnosis of necrotizing enterocolitis (NEC).[55] This chapter was demonstrated as a novel method of abdominal infrared thermal imaging that is capable of intestinal inflammation characteristics of NEC. The result hopefully suggested that this new noncontact, nonionizing method could be used as an early diagnostic tool.[55]

8.5 CONCLUSION AND FUTURE DIRECTIONS

IRT is an innovative method for studying body surface temperature and tissue perfusion in adults, children, and newborns in both research and clinical settings. This technique is noninvasive and convenient (due to advancement in sensor technology) and does not expose neonates to hazardous radiation. The potential for new research with infrared imaging is growing rapidly. For example, nursing researchers can use thermography to monitor wounds and identify skin temperature variations associated with pressure injuries, as the temperature differential between normal skin and skin that is deteriorating due to infection can be detected long before visual examination reveals discoloration as a result of impaired skin integrity.

Neonatal researchers can apply this technology in a variety of areas, including studying kangaroo care, which involves the transfer of heat between the mother's breast and the wrapped baby, cooling the body for hypoxic–ischemic encephalopathy treatment, and NEC.

In NICU, body temperature, ECG, respiratory rate, and blood oxygen saturation are the primary vital indicators of clinical significance for continuous neonatal monitoring. Presently, in the neonates, the body temperature is measured by the adhesive thermistor and also ECG; RR is measured by adhesive skin electrodes. The placement and removal of these adhesive skin sensors (electrodes) and the presence of all wire are discomforts and even painful stimuli. Accordingly, the most important cause of skin breakdown is removal of sticky electrodes from newborns in intensive care units. Hence, an alternative, noninvasive, noncontact method is needed for the monitoring of vital physiological function to provide neonatal care and monitoring. The thermal imaging has demonstrated the potential for accurate temperature and respiratory detection. However, there are still many challenges and concrete pieces of evidence needed in terms of clinical evaluation.

IRT-based innovation has the potential to reduce neonatal therapeutic costs and length of stay for newborns who have illness like NEC or hypoperfusion, or who have surgery to fix a problem with their stomachs. This innovation is in its earliest stages, and chances for research abound. As researchers continue to study this prospective technique, they will uncover a variety of other research and therapeutic applications.

In the future, thermal image-based monitoring is not limited to neonatal monitoring but is also used for high-risk patients during the critical operating phase. For that, a lot of research work, clinical trials, and case studies are needed to make it feasible for life risk. Thermal imaging represents a new era in medical research with a bright future.

KEYWORDS

- **infrared thermography**
- **neonatal monitoring**
- **medical diagnosis**

REFERENCES

1. Maurya, L.; Kaur, P.; Chawla, D.; Mahapatra, P. Non-contact Breathing Rate Monitoring in Newborns: A Review. *Comput. Biol. Med.* **2021,** *132*, 104321. DOI: 10.1016/j.compbiomed.2021.104321.
2. Millennium Development Goals (MDGs). https://www.who.int/news-room/fact-sheets/detail/millennium-development-goals-(mdgs), 15-3-2021.
3. Abbas, A. K.; Heimann, K.; Blazek, V.; Orlikowsky, T.; Leonhardt, S. Neonatal Infrared Thermography Imaging: Analysis of Heat Flux During Different Clinical Scenarios. *Infrared Phys. Technol.* **2012,** *55* (6), 538–548. DOI: 10.1016/j.infrared.2012.07.001.
4. World Health Organization. *Thermal Protection of the Newborn: A Practical Guide*; World Health Organization, 1997.
5. Pereira, C. B.; Yu, X.; Goos, T.; Reiss, I.; Orlikowsky, T.; Heimann, K.; Venema, B.; Blazek, V.; Leonhardt, S.; Teichmann, D. Noncontact Monitoring of Respiratory Rate in Newborn Infants Using Thermal Imaging. *IEEE Trans. Biomed. Eng.* **2019,** *66* (4), 1105–1114. DOI: 10.1109/TBME.2018.2866878.
6. Hasan, M.; Negulescu, I. Wearable Technology for Baby Monitoring: A Review. *J. Text. Eng. Fashion Technol.* **2020,** *6* (4), 112–120.
7. Bouwstra, S.; Chen, W.; Feijs, L.; Oetomo, S. B. Smart Jacket Design for Neonatal Monitoring with Wearable Sensors. In *2009 Sixth International Workshop on Wearable and Implantable Body Sensor Networks*; 2009. DOI: 10.1109/BSN.2009.40.
8. Sato, S.; Ishida-Nakajima, W.; Ishida, A.; Kawamura, M.; Miura, S.; Ono, K.; Inagaki, N.; Takada, G.; Takahashi, T. Assessment of a New Piezoelectric Transducer Sensor for Noninvasive Cardiorespiratory Monitoring of Newborn Infants in the NICU. *Neonatology* **2010,** *98* (2), 179–190. DOI: 10.1159/000283994.
9. Kraaijenga, J. V.; Hutten, G. J.; de Jongh, F. H.; van Kaam, A. H. Transcutaneous Electromyography of the Diaphragm: A Cardio-Respiratory Monitor for Preterm Infants. *Pediatr. Pulmonol.* **2015,** *50* (9), 889–895. DOI: 10.1002/ppul.23116.
10. Joshi, R.; Bierling, B.; Feijs, L.; van Pul, C.; Andriessen, P. Monitoring the Respiratory Rate of Preterm Infants Using an Ultrathin Film Sensor Embedded in the Bedding: A Comparative Feasibility Study. *Physiol. Meas.* **2019,** *40* (4), 045003. DOI: 10.1088/1361-6579/ab1595.
11. Raj, A. A.; et al. Clinical Validation of a Wearable Respiratory Rate Device for Neonatal Monitoring. In *2018 40th Annual International Conference of the IEEE Engineering in Medicine and Biology Society (EMBC)*; 2018.

12. Zhu, Z.; Liu, T.; Li, G.; Li, T.; Inoue, Y. Wearable Sensor Systems for Infants. *Sensors (Basel)* **2015,** *15* (2), 3721–3749. DOI: 10.3390/s150203721.
13. Knobel, R. B.; Guenther, B. D.; Rice, H. E. Thermoregulation and Thermography in Neonatal Physiology and Disease. *Biol. Res. Nurs.* **2011,** *13* (3), 274–282. DOI: 10.1177/1099800411403467.
14. Pereira, C. B.; Yu, X.; Czaplik, M.; Rossaint, R.; Blazek, V.; Leonhardt, S. Remote Monitoring of Breathing Dynamics Using Infrared Thermography. *Biomed. Opt. Express* **2015,** *6* (11), 4378–4394. DOI: 10.1364/BOE.6.004378.
15. Maurya, L.; Mahapatra, P.; Chawla, D. Non-contact Breathing Monitoring by Integrating RGB and Thermal Imaging via RGB-Thermal Image Registration. *Biocybern. Biomed. Eng.* **2021,** *41* (3), 1107–1122. DOI: 10.1016/j.bbe.2021.07.002.
16. Droitcour, A. D.; Seto, T. B.; Park, B. K.; Yamada, S.; Vergara, A.; El Hourani, C.; Shing, T.; Yuen, A.; Lubecke, V. M.; Boric-Lubecke, O. Non-contact Respiratory Rate Measurement Validation for Hospitalized Patients. In EMBC *2009. Annual International Conference of the IEEE*, Engineering in Medicine and Biology Society; IEEE: New York, NY, 2009. DOI: 10.1109/IEMBS.2009.5332635.
17. Bartula, M.; Tigges, T.; Muehlsteff, J. Camera-Based System for Contactless Monitoring of Respiration. In *35th Annual International Conference of the IEEE*, Engineering in Medicine and Biology Society (EMBC); IEEE: New York, NY, 2013. DOI: 10.1109/EMBC.2013.6610090.
18. van Gastel, M.; Stuijk, S.; de Haan, G. Robust Respiration Detection from Remote Photoplethysmography. *Biomed. Opt. Express* **2016,** *7* (12), 4941–4957. DOI: 10.1364/BOE.7.004941.
19. Lahiri, B. B.; Bagavathiappan, S.; Jayakumar, T.; Philip, J. Medical Applications of Infrared Thermography: A Review. *Infrared Phys. Technol.* **2012,** *55* (4), 221–235. DOI: 10.1016/j.infrared.2012.03.007.
20. Herschel, W. Investigation of the Powers of the Prismatic Colours to Heat and Illuminate Objects, with Remarks That Prove the Different Refrangibility of Radiant Heat. To Which Is Added, an Inquiry into the Method of Viewing the Sun Advantageously, with Telescopes of Large Apertures and High Magnifying Powers. By William Herschel, LL. *DFRS. Philos. Trans. R. Soc. Lond.* **1800,** *90*, 255–283.
21. Ring, E. F. J. The Historical Development of Temperature Measurement in Medicine. *Infrared Phys. Technol.* **2007,** *49* (3), 297–301. DOI: 10.1016/j.infrared.2006.06.029.
22. Lawson, R. Implications of Surface Temperatures in the Diagnosis of Breast Cancer. *Can. Med. Assoc. J.* **1956,** *75* (4), 309–311.
23. Jones, B. F. A Reappraisal of the Use of Infrared Thermal Image Analysis in Medicine. *IEEE Trans. Med. Imaging* **1998,** *17* (6), 1019–1027. DOI: 10.1109/42.746635.
24. Steketee, J. Spectral Emissivity of Skin and Pericardium. *Phys. Med. Biol.* **1973,** *18* (5), 686–694. DOI: 10.1088/0031-9155/18/5/307.
25. Handbook of Infrared Detection Technologies. In *Handbook of Infrared Detection Technologies*; Vol. III; Elsevier Science: Amsterdam; p 2002.
26. Williams, T. *An Introduction to Thermal Imaging, Thermal Imaging Cameras*; CRC Press: Boca Raton, FL, 2009.
27. Vainer, B. *The Use of Infrared Thermography for Investigation of Thermoregulation in Humans. Body Temperature Regulation*; Nova Science Publishers Inc.: New York, NY, 2009.

28. Miller, L. M.; Smith, R. J. Synchrotrons Versus Globars, Point-Detectors Versus Focal Plane Arrays: Selecting the Best Source and Detector for Specific Infrared Microspectroscopy and Imaging Applications. *Vib. Spectrosc.* **2005,** *38* (1), 237–240.
29. Qi, H.; Diakides, N. A. *Infrared Imaging in Medicine*; CRC Press: Boca Raton, FL, 2007.
30. Bagavathiappan, S.; Saravanan, T.; Philip, J.; Jayakumar, T.; Raj, B.; Karunanithi, R.; Panicker, T. M.; Korath, M. P.; Jagadeesan, K. Infrared Thermal Imaging for Detection of Peripheral Vascular Disorders. *J. Med. Phys.* **2009,** *34* (1), 43–47. DOI: 10.4103/0971-6203.48720.
31. Bharara, M.; Cobb, J. E.; Claremont, D. J. Thermography and Thermometry in the Assessment of Diabetic Neuropathic Foot: A Case for Furthering the Role of Thermal Techniques. *Int. J. Low. Extrem. Wounds* **2006,** *5* (4), 250–260. DOI: 10.1177/1534734 606293481.
32. Mercer, J. B.; Nielsen, S. P.; Hoffmann, G. Improvement of Wound Healing by Water-Filtered Infrared-A (wIRA) in Patients with Chronic Venous Stasis Ulcers of the Lower Legs Including Evaluation Using Infrared Thermography. *Ger. Med. Sci.* **2008,** *6*, Doc11.
33. Mital, M.; Scott, E. P. Thermal Detection of Embedded Tumors Using Infrared Imaging. *J. Biomech. Eng.* **2007,** *129* (1), 33–39. DOI: 10.1115/1.2401181.
34. Nakanishi, R.; Imai-Matsumura, K. Facial Skin Temperature Decreases in Infants with Joyful Expression. *Infant Behav. Dev.* **2008,** *31* (1), 137–144. DOI: 10.1016/j.infbeh.2007.09.001.
35. Akio, N.; Munecazu, T. Correlation Analysis on Alpha Attenuation and Nasal Skin Temperature. *J. Stat. Mech. Theor. Exp.* **2009,** *01*, 01007.
36. Hammarlund, K.; Strömberg, B.; Sedin, G. Heat Loss from the Skin of Preterm and Fullterm Newborn Infants during the First Weeks After Birth. *Biol. Neonate* **1986,** *50* (1), 1–10. DOI: 10.1159/000242554.
37. Stolwijk, J. A. Heat Exchangers between Body and Environment. *Bibl. Radiol.* **1975,** *1975* (6), 144–150.
38. Helmy, A.; Holdmann, M.; Rizkalla, M. Application of Thermography for Non-invasive Diagnosis of Thyroid Gland Disease. *IEEE Trans. Bio Med. Eng.* **2008,** *55* (3), 1168–1175. DOI: 10.1109/TBME.2008.915731.
39. Charkoudian, N. Mechanisms and Modifiers of Reflex Induced Cutaneous Vasodilation and Vasoconstriction in Humans. *J. Appl. Physiol. (1985)* **2010,** *109* (4), 1221–1228. DOI: 10.1152/japplphysiol.00298.2010.
40. Pereira, C. B.; Czaplik, M.; Blanik, N.; Rossaint, R.; Blazek, V.; Leonhardt, S. Contact-Free Monitoring of Circulation and Perfusion Dynamics Based on the Analysis of Thermal Imagery. *Biomed. Opt. Express* **2014,** *5* (4), 1075–1089. DOI: 10.1364/BOE.5.001075.
41. Chiang, M. F.; Lin, P. W.; Lin, L. F.; Chiou, H. Y.; Chien, C. W.; Chu, S. F.; Chiu, W. T. Mass Screening of Suspected Febrile Patients with Remote-Sensing Infrared Thermography: Alarm Temperature and Optimal Distance. *J. Formos. Med. Assoc.* **2008,** *107* (12), 937–944. DOI: 10.1016/S0929-6646(09)60017-6.
42. Chiu, W. T.; Lin, P. W.; Chiou, H. Y.; Lee, W. S.; Lee, C. N.; Yang, Y. Y.; Lee, H. M.; Hsieh, M. S.; Hu, C. J.; Ho, Y. S.; Deng, W. P.; Hsu, C. Y. Infrared Thermography to

Mass-Screen Suspected SARS Patients with Fever. *Asia Pac. J. Public Health* **2005,** *17* (1), 26–28. DOI: 10.1177/101053950501700107.
43. Goetz, C.; Foertsch, D.; Schoenberger, J.; Uhl, E. Thermography—A Valuable Tool to Test Hydrocephalus Shunt Patency. *Acta Neurochir.* **2005,** *147* (11), 1167–1172; discussion 1172. DOI: 10.1007/s00701-005-0608-1.
44. Merla, A.; Mattei, P. A.; Di Donato, L.; Romani, G. L. Thermal Imaging of Cutaneous Temperature Modifications in Runners During Graded Exercise. *Ann. Biomed. Eng.* **2010,** *38* (1), 158–163. DOI: 10.1007/s10439-009-9809-8.
45. Barnes, R. B. Thermography of the Human Body. *Science* **1963,** *140* (3569), 870–877. DOI: 10.1126/science.140.3569.870.
46. Clark, R. P.; Stothers, J. K. Neonatal Skin Temperature Distribution Using Infra-Red Colour Thermography. *J. Physiol.* **1980,** *302*, 323–333. DOI: 10.1113/jphysiol.1980.sp013245.
47. Anderson, E. S.; Wailoo, M. P.; Petersen, S. A. Use of Thermographic Imaging to Study Babies Sleeping at Home. *Arch. Dis. Child.* **1990,** *65* (11), 1266–1267. DOI: 10.1136/adc.65.11.1266.
48. Rylander, E. V. A.; Přibylová, H.; Lind, J. A Thermographic Study of Infants Exposed to Cold. *Acta Paediatr.* **1972,** *61* (1), 42–48. DOI: 10.1111/j.1651-2227.1972.tb15901.x.
49. Adams, A. K.; Nelson, R. A.; Bell, E. F.; Egoavil, C. A. Use of Infrared Thermographic Calorimetry to Determine Energy Expenditure in Preterm Infants. *Am. J. Clin. Nutr.* **2000,** *71* (4), 969–977. DOI: 10.1093/ajcn/71.4.969.
50. Christidis, I.; Zotter, H.; Rosegger, H.; Engele, H.; Kurz, R.; Kerbl, R. Infrared Thermography in Newborns: The First Hour After Birth. *Gynäkol. Geburtshilfliche Rundsch.* **2003,** *43* (1), 31–35. DOI: 10.1159/000067168.
51. Heimann, K.; Jergus, K.; Abbas, A. K.; Heussen, N.; Leonhardt, S.; Orlikowsky, T. Infrared Thermography for Detailed Registration of Thermoregulation in Premature Infants. *J. Perinat. Med.* **2013,** *41* (5), 613–620. DOI: 10.1515/jpm-2012-0239.
52. Abbas, A. K.; Heimann, K.; Jergus, K.; Orlikowsky, T.; Leonhardt, S. Neonatal Non-contact Respiratory Monitoring Based on Real-Time Infrared Thermography. *Biomed. Eng. Online* **2011,** *10* (1), 93. DOI: 10.1186/1475-925X-10-93.
53. Klaessens, J.; et al. Development of a Baby Friendly Noncontact Method for Measuring Vital Signs: First Results of Clinical Measurements in an Open Incubator at a Neonatal Intensive Care Unit. In *SPIE Bios*; SPIE, 2014; Vol. 8935.
54. Pereira, C. B.; Heimann, K.; Venema, B.; Blazek, V.; Czaplik, M.; Leonhardt, S. Estimation of Respiratory Rate from Thermal Videos of Preterm Infants. Conference Proceedings. *Annu. Int. Conf. IEEE Eng. Med. Biol. Soc.* **2017,** *2017*, 3818–3821. DOI: 10.1109/EMBC.2017.8037689.
55. Ourselin, S.; et al. Image Processing of Infrared Thermal Images for the Detection of Necrotizing Enterocolitis. *Med. Imaging Image Process* **2013,** *2013*.

CHAPTER 9

Retinal Disease Diagnosis Using Machine Learning Techniques

G. KALAIARASI[1], B. SARITHA[2], S. K. KABILESH[2], and D. MOHANAPRIYA[2]

[1]*Department of ACSE, Vignan Foundation for Science, Technology and Research, Andhra Pradesh, India*

[2]*Jai Shriram Engineering College, Tirupur, Tamil Nadu, India*

ABSTRACT

The retinal cells play a crucial role in vision. An electric signal is converted into light signals by the retina and sent to the brain. The most common diseases in the retina are diabetic retinopathy and glaucoma. In this chapter, retinal diseases are detected using an image-processing technique. Due to increased intraocular pressure within the eye, optical nerves become damaged, which results in glaucoma. Having diabetes for more than 20 years leads to diabetic retinopathy, which leads to damage to the retina. Glaucoma was detected using the cup-to-disc ratio and diabetic retinopathy was detected using a gray-level co-occurrence matrix. By using the support vector machine (SVM) classifier, retinal diseases are detected efficiently with 92.3% accuracy. Retinal disease detection includes three main parts: preprocessing, feature extraction, and classification. In the preprocessing part, a green channel is extracted which is followed by a top-hat filter transformation. It is used to improve the contrast between the region of interest and the foreground. Edge detection is performed by the median filter and the Gaussian filter is used to remove noise. With the preprocessed image, the texture-based and color-based features are extracted for classification. Finally, retinal diseases are detected by training the SVM classifier.

Applied Intelligence for Medical Image Analysis. Aarti, Raju Pal, Mukesh Saraswat, & Himanshu Mittal (Eds.)

9.1 INTRODUCTION

9.1.1 DIABETIC RETINOPATHY

This disease comes based on blood sugar levels. This can cause vision loss and blindness. If anyone is affected by diabetes, a person must consult an ophthalmologist once a year. Too much sugar in the blood can damage the retina. It does not have any symptoms at the starting stage, but early detection can help to take steps to protect our vision. The tiny blood vessels go to the retina and make blood blocks. This may cause very severe effects on the eyes. The diameter and width variations in the vessels that represent managing the blood sugar level will decrease diabetic retinopathy (DR). To overcome DR eating healthy, physical activity and carefully following the doctors' instructions for insulin or diabetics medicine. Diabetes and high blood pressure will increase the risk of DR. The later symptoms of DR are blurry vision, difficulty in reading, and floating spots in vision. The sensitive layer of tissue is the retina and it is easily affected by DR. Figure 9.1 shows the comparison of DR-affected retina and normal retina.

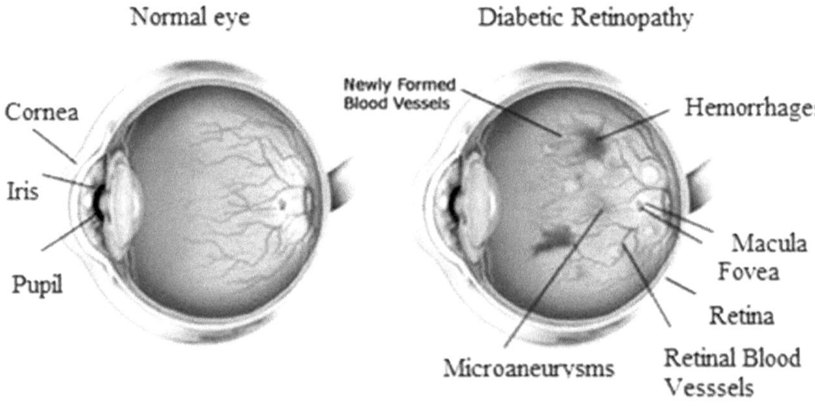

FIGURE 9.1 Comparison of DR-affected retina and normal retina.

Image courtesy: Manhattan Eye Specialists. https://www.eyedoctorophthalmologistnyc.com/treatment/diabetic-retinopathy-eye-disease/

9.1.2 GLAUCOMA

The eye disease glaucoma can cause loss of vision. Glaucoma disease damages the optic nerves in the back of the eye. There is no solution for glaucoma. Only early detection of glaucoma can help protect our vision. Open-angle glaucoma is one of the main types of glaucoma. Similar to DR, glaucoma also does not have any symptoms at the starting stage. However, at a severe stage, the loss of side vision and blindness are the symptoms. Laser treatment and eye drops are the initial stage treatments. Surgery is the last treatment to protect the vision. The size of the normal optic disc and disease-affected retina is shown in Figure 9.2.

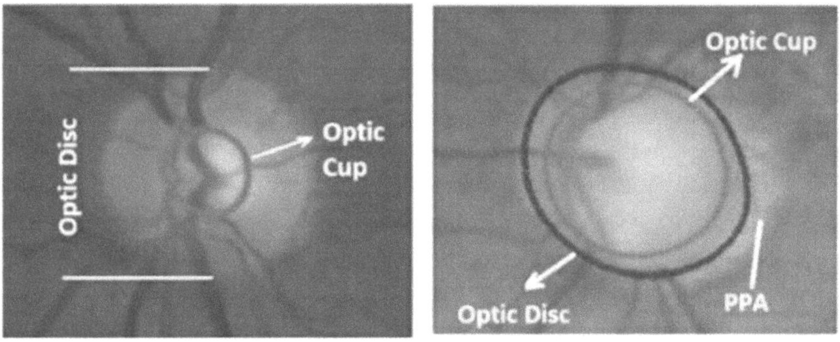

FIGURE 9.2 Optic disc of normal retina and glaucoma-affected retina.

9.2 LITERATURE SURVEY

The automatic detection of retinal diseases has been proposed in many related works. A vertical cup-to-disc ratio (VCDR) of an image is determined by the height of the optic disc and the cup. This resulted in a weighted VCDR mean difference of 0.11. The optic disc and cup are estimated with the help of relative height error.[1] Color and texture features are extracted from the fundus image of the blood vessels. Before feature extraction, noisy pixels are eliminated. A retinal fundus image can be characterized clinically by using features such as color and texture extracted from it. These features are fed into the SVM artificial neural networks (ANN) for further classification.[2,15,21]

Several computer-based algorithms have been proposed for the detection of glaucoma. Most of the existing methods focus on the calculation of the cup-to-disc ratio (CDR), but they fail to consider the size of the optical disc (OD) because the size of the OD differs from person to person.[3]

Deep convolutional neural networks are implemented to identify the presence of exudates and thereby classify it into DR or cataract.[4] Bright lesions on the retina are one of the symptoms of DR detected by an automatic DR detection system. A fundus image is constructed by first removing the optic disc. A variety of features are extracted from exudates. For the detection of different stages of the disease, random forest algorithms and ANN were used.[5] From the fundus image, the optic disc was identified to separate the retinal damaged vascular tissues. Two types of lesions are present in damaged areas. The presence of dark lesions is used to detect various stages of DR.[6]

DR infection level is found through the detection of two essential types of DRs; hemorrhages and exudates. Using fundus pictures of patients and appropriately preparing these fundus pictures can remove these sorts of problems. Using these sorts and their sum in the fundus images, the level of DR in the patient will be determined.[7] Preprocessing, such as removing noise and improving image quality, is incorporated in the proposed method. The image features are extracted using principle component analysis and the extracted features are classified using SVM for classification. These methods provided effective classification techniques for fundus images.[8]

To extract features from an image, an initial stage of image processing isolates blood vessels, micro-aneurysms, and hard exudates. An SVM classifier was used to train these features to detect DR.[9] After the initial enhancement of the image is performed using the preprocessing stage, curvelet transforms are applied to the equalized image. The blood vessels are extracted from the enhanced image.

From blood vessels and optic disc extracted images, exudates were estimated using better PSNR.[10,20] The exudates were detected to find the presence of diabetic macular edema. An analysis of the color and wavelet decomposition features of a fundus retinal image is performed.[11,17] Automated OD localization in retinal images was used to locate the OD and its center on all retinal images. The algorithm in this chapter provided excellent results and avoided false optic disc detection.[12] The circular Hough transform and convolution neural network algorithms were combined for detecting exudates.[13,16] Segmentation using a deep neural network trained on large images, preprocessed with global contrast normalization, zero-phase whitening, and augmented with geometric transformations and gamma correction.[14,18] Structured prediction uses a network to simultaneously classify multiple pixels.

9.3 EXISTING METHOD

The blind spot is located using COSFIRE (combination of shifted filter responses) filters. The fundus image is applied to the COSFIRE filter. Detection of divergent points in the major vessels in the retina is done with the vasculature selective filter. The large region was cropped by this filter. In this population-based glaucoma screening, eight public dataset collections are manually annotated by an accomplished ophthalmologist. In the methodology, the first step is to restrict the vulnerable side by utilizing two sorts of teachable COSFIRE channels: one designed to be particular to the different localities of vessel trees, and another arranged to be specific to roundabout brilliant areas. Then, at that point, fit a circle that approximates the limit of the distinguished optic plate. Then, summed-up lattice learning vector quantization was applied to section the portrayed vulnerable side into two districts: the cup and the neuroretinal edge. At last, figure out the VCDR and supply an unwavering quality score of the estimation. The plate-specific COSFIRE channel identifies the splendid circle examples and harvests the little area around the most extreme reaction of this channel. The recognized optic plate is fitted around like a circle. To portion the plate area into the neuroretinal edge and the cup, summed up, lattice learning vector quantization is utilized. The blue limit inside the plate is still up in the air cup. As a result, the VCDR was calculated based on the determined cup and disc to yield a reliability score.

9.4 PROPOSED METHOD

DR and glaucoma are performed using image-processing techniques. The first step involves preprocessing. It includes contrast enhancement, green channel extraction, noise removal by filters, and intensity adjustment. The texture-based features are extracted from the preprocessed image.

SVM classifiers are used for classification. These features are used to train, test, and validate the SVM classifier. Fundus datasets are collected from eye hospitals situated locally. For more accuracy, some standard datasets were collected from the Online Retinal Fundus Image database for Glaucoma Analysis and Research. A total of 150 images were collected for DIARETDB1 (Diabetic Retinopathy DataBase calibration level 1) and MESSIDOR (Method to Evaluate Segmentation and Indexing Techniques in Retinal Ophthalmology) standards, 75 images were trained, 25 images were tested, and 25 images were validated.

TABLE 9.1 Feature Extraction from the Fundus Image.

Feature	Description
Mean	Each plane's average pixel value
Standard deviation	The variance distribution measure
Variance	The average squared difference between pixel intensities
Skewness	Measure the asymmetry of the color distribution
Entropy	Tests for randomness
Energy	The uniformity of pixel intensities is measured

9.4.1 PREPROCESSING

The first step is to preprocess the fundus images, by using the standard datasets. The collected datasets have different resolutions. For image resizing, a standard 1500 × 1500 resolution range is used. The green channel is extracted from a RGB image as part of the preprocessing technique as shown in Figure 9.3. It is followed by steps such as inversion and contrast enhancement. Gaussian filters are used to remove the noise from the fundus image. The brightness of the optic disc is enhanced by using a top-hat filter. For edge detection of an image, median filters are used. Then, the background is removed for better efficiency. During preprocessing, intensities are adjusted to increase contrast.

9.4.2 FEATURE EXTRACTION

In order to detect glaucoma, optic CDR is considered. Using the green component threshold value, the OD is extracted from the retinal image. The diameter of the optic disc and optic cup was determined to evaluate the CDR. An image's CDR can be defined as the ratio of a cup portion to a disc portion. A region's centroid, major axis length, minor axis length, diameter, and radius are calculated. Subtracting the disc area from the cup area of the image yields the rim area. Then, the rim-to-disc ratio (RDR) is determined. The RDR is defined as the ratio of the rim area to the disc area of an image:

$$\text{CDR} = \frac{\text{Area of cup}}{\text{Area of disc}} \frac{\text{Area of cup}}{\text{Area of disc}} \tag{9.1}$$

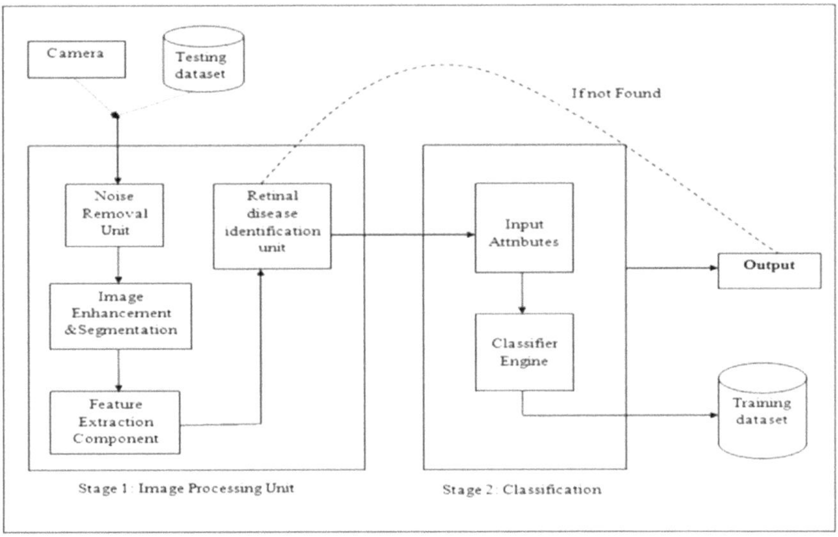

FIGURE 9.3 Block diagram.

For DR detection, blood vessels are extracted using the threshold value. Edge detection is done by converting the vessel-extracted image into a binary image. To train the SVM classifier, texture-based features such as the GLCM (gray-level co-occurrence matrix) are extracted from that binary image. By analyzing spatial relationships among pixels, it is a statistical way of examining texture. GLCM feature extraction determines factors such as energy, entropy, homogeneity, contrast, and correlation. Several color-based features are calculated, including mean, variance, standard deviation, and entropy. Color features extracted from the fundus image are given in Table 9.1. The linear classifier is defined as

$$f(x) = W^T X + bf(x) = W^T X + b \tag{9.2}$$

W and b represent weight and bias, respectively. Weighing and biasing are represented by W and b, respectively. For DR detection, blood vessels are extracted using the threshold value. Edge detection is done by converting the vessel-extracted image into a binary image. From that binary image, texture-based features like GLCM are extracted to train the SVM classifier.

A statistical method of analyzing texture considers pixels' spatial relationship. In GLCM feature extraction, factors like energy, entropy, homogeneity, contrast, and correlation are determined. Color-based features like mean, variance, standard deviation, entropy, and energy are determined. Glaucoma-affected image is shown in Figure 9.4.

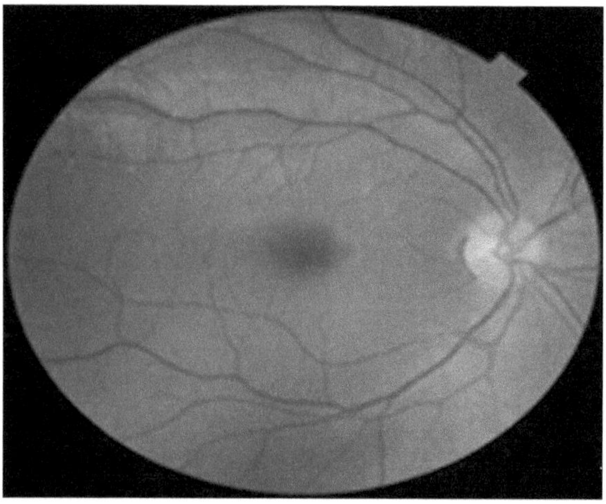

FIGURE 9.4 Input glaucoma image.

Source: Adapted from Ref. [22]. http://creativecommons.org/licenses/by/4.0/

9.4.3 CLASSIFICATION

Classification is done by an SVM classifier. The fundus retina is classified as normal or abnormal using this supervised learning method. If it is an abnormal image, then it is again classified into glaucoma or DR-affected image. After the feature extraction classification process, there are two important tasks, that is, training and testing sets. The datasets are separated into these two sets. There are several attributes and three targets. An attribute is a feature extracted from the preprocessing of the fundus image. The target is the output, whether the fundus image is glaucoma or DR affected the image or normal image. The SVM classifier shows excellent performance in the field of pattern recognition. The attributes collected from the preprocessing techniques serve as test data. Only small training is needed for the SVM classifier to provide better performance. And it needs a few minutes of runtime for training purposes. The computational efficiency is greater in the SVM classifier. The advantage is that the SVM classifier provides efficient datasets and it gives results with an accuracy rate of 92.3% and sensitivity of 100%. The evaluated confusion matrix is shown in Figure 9.5.

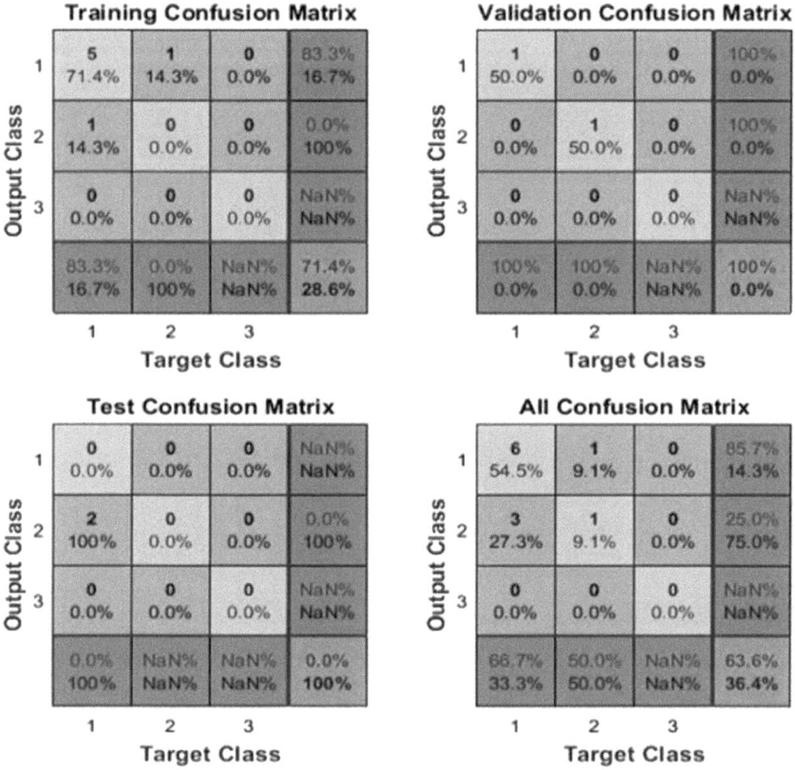

FIGURE 9.5 Confusion matrix for training, test, validation, and overall.

9.5 RESULT

Features like micro-aneurysm area, entropy, correlation, and energy are obtained from the preprocessed fundus image. These features are provided as input to the SVM classifier. This technique is implemented using MatLab. More than 75 images were processed to extract texture-based and color-based features. Twenty-five images are considered normal eye fundus images, 25 are glaucoma images, and 25 are DR images. An input image is given to the SVM classifier; it gives the gradient image as represented in Figure 9.6. After gradient feature extraction, the DR-affected part alone was extracted by the SVM classifier shown in Figure 9.7. In Figure 9.8, glaucoma-affected parts are shown in red color and other areas in blue dots.

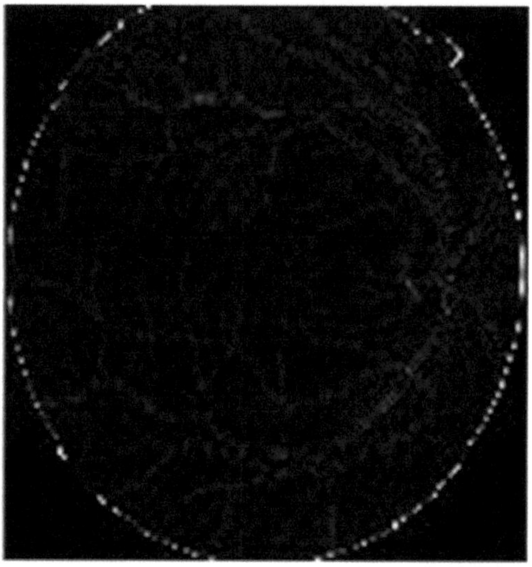

FIGURE 9.6 Gradient image.

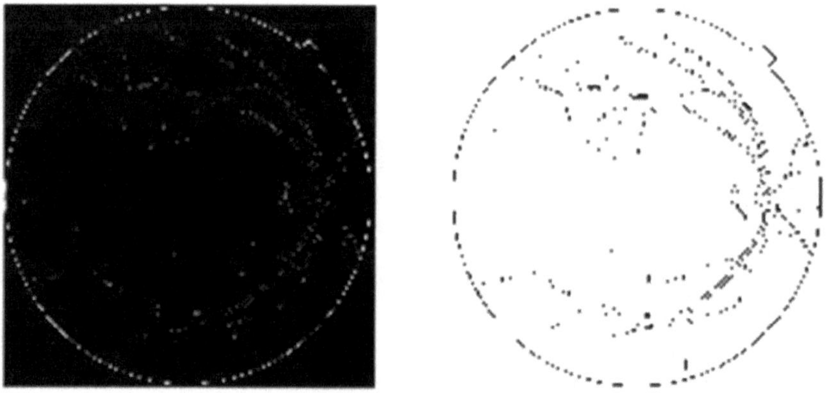

FIGURE 9.7 Glaucoma extraction using SVM.

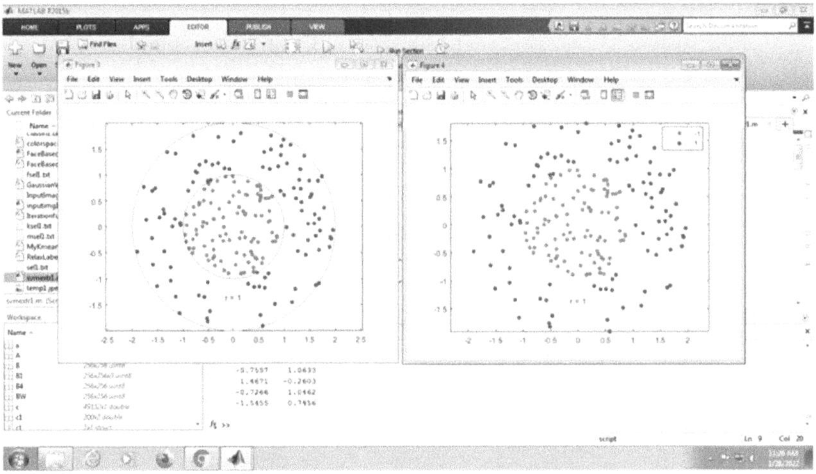

FIGURE 9.8 Support vector machine kernel trick for classification.

9.6 CONCLUSION

Glaucoma and DR result in blindness. Early detection and diagnosis are necessary for prediagnosis of vision loss. This chapter gives the design and implementation for detecting the presence of retinal diseases like glaucoma and DR. The retinal fundus image is preprocessed to extract the texture-based and color-based features. Using the extracted features, an SVM classifier is trained to distinguish disease-affected retinas from normal retinas. In addition, the SVM classifier provides 92.3% accuracy in detecting retinal diseases. It is easy to extend this approach to detect multiple types of diseases in fundus images.

9.7 FUTURE SCOPE

Future work includes a detailed analysis of retinal disease detection. The method can be tested with more datasets which gives more accuracy. One possible approach could be expanding the analysis of more diseases that affect the retina like a macular hole and macular degeneration. An alternative approach is to modify the entire process to determine the presence of glaucoma and DR. Glaucoma can be determined by using the inferior–superior–nasal–temporal ratio.

KEYWORDS

- **blood sugar levels**
- **diabetics medicine**
- **glaucoma**
- **optic disc**
- **retinal fundus**

REFERENCES

1. Guo, J.; Azzopardi, G.; et al. Automatic Determination of Vertical Cup-to-Disc Ratio in Retinal Fundus Images for Glaucoma Screening. *IEEE Access* **2019,** *4*. DOI: 10.1109/Access.2018.2890544.
2. Pathan, S.; Kumar, P.; Pai, R. M. The Role of Color and Texture Features in Glaucoma Detection. In *IEEE Conference*, 2018. DOI: 10.1109/ICACCI.2018.8554854.
3. Thakur, N.; Juneja, M. Survey on Segmentation and Classification Approaches of Optic Cup and Optic Disc for Diagnosis of Glaucoma. *Biomed. Signal Process. Control* **2018,** *42*, 162–189. DOI: 10.1016/J.BSPC.2018.01.014.
4. Kazi, A.; Ajmera, M.; Sukhija, P.; Devadkar, K. Processing Retinal Images to Discover Diseases. In *IEEE International Conference on Current Trends toward Converging Technologies*, 2018. DOI: 10.1109/ICCTCT.2018.8550942.
5. Prabhu, N.; Bhoir, D.; Shanbhag, N. Diabetic Retinopathy Screening Using Machine Learning for Hierarchical Classification. *Int. J. Innov. Technol. Explor. Eng. (IJITEE)* **2019,** *8* (10, August). ISSN: 2278-3075
6. Shetty, S.; Kari, K. B.; Rathod, J. A. Detection of Diabetic Retinopathy Using Support Vector Machine. *Int. J. Emerg. Technol. Comput. Sci. Electron. (IJETCSE)* **2016,** 23 (6). ISSN: 0976-1353.
7. Ramya, V. SVM Based Detection for Diabetic Retinopathy. *Int. J. Res. Sci. Innov.* **2018,** *V* (I). ISSN 2321–2705.
8. AbhishekDey; Bandyopadhyay, S. K. Automated Glaucoma Detection Using Support Vector Machine Classification Method. *Br. J. Med. Med. Res.* **2016,** *11* (12). ISSN: 2231-0614.
9. Carrera, E. V.; Gonzalez, A.; Carrera, R. Automated Detection of Diabetic Retinopathy Using SVM. In *Conference Paper*, August 2017. DOI: 10.1109/INTERCON.2017.8079692.
10. Singh, B.; Jayasree, K. Implementation of Diabetic Retinopathy Detection System for Enhance Digital Fundus Images. *Int. J. Adv. Technol. Innov. Res.* **2015,** *7* (6), 874–876.
11. Giancardo, L.; Meriaudeau, F.; Karnowski, T. P.; et al. Exudates-Based Diabetic Macular Edema Detection in Fundus Images Using Publicly Available Datasets. *Med. Image Anal.* **2012,** *16*, 216–226.

12. Godse, D. A.; Bormane, D. S. Automated Localization of Optic Disc in Retinal Images. *IJACSA* **2013,** *4* (2). DOI: 10.14569/IJACSA.2013.040210.
13. Adem, K. *Exudate Detection for Diabetic Retinopathy with Circular Hough Transformation and Convolutional Neural Networks*; Elsevier Ltd: Amsterdam, 2018. DOI: 10.1016/J.ESWA.2018.07.053.
14. Liskowski, P.; Krawiec, K. Segmenting Retinal Blood Vessels with Deep Neural Networks. *IEEE Trans. Med. Imaging* **2016,** *35* (11), 2369–2380. DOI: 10.1109/TMI.2016.2546227.
15. Kabilesh, S. K.; Revathi, K.; Sabitha, K.; Sujithkumar, N. Medical Image Counterfeit Detection for Smart Healthcare. *J. Sens. Res. Technol.* **2020,** *2* (2), 1–6.
16. Sagayaraj, A. S.; Kabilesh, S. K.; Kumar, A. A.; Gokulnath, S.; Mani, T.; Dinakaran, K. Diabetes Mellitus and Diabetic Retinopathy Detection Using Tongue Images. *J. Phys. Conf. Ser.* **2021,** *1831* (1), 012028. DOI: 10.1088/1742-6596/1831/1/012028.
17. Kumar, A. A.; Mani, T.; Gokulnath, S.; Kabilesh, S. K.; Dinakaran, K.; Sagayaraj, A. S. Screening of Tuberculosis Using Artificial Neural Network. *Int. J. Res. Eng. Sci. Manage.* **2020,** *3* (11), 145–149.
18. Kalaiarasi, G.; Maheswari, S. Deep Proximal Support Vector Machine Classifiers for Hyperspectral Images Classification. *Neural Comput. Appl.* **2021,** *33* (20), 13391–13415. DOI: 10.1007/s00521-021-05965-0.
19. Balasubramaniyan, S.; Jeyakumar, V.; Nachimuthu, D. S. Panoramic Tongue Imaging and Deep Convolutional Machine Learning Model for Diabetes Diagnosis in Humans. *Sci. Rep.* **2022,** *12* (1). DOI: 10.1038/s41598-021-03879-4.
20. Sagayaraj, A. S.; Kabilesh, S. K.; Mohanapriya, D.; Anandkumar, A. Determination of Soil Moisture Content Using Image Processing—A Survey. In *2021 6th International Conference on Inventive Computation Technologies (ICICT)*, 2021; pp 1101–1106. DOI: 10.1109/ICICT50816.2021.9358736.
21. Ramya, G.; Janarthanan, P. P.; Mohanapriya, D. Steganography Based Data Hiding for Security Applications. In *2018 International Conference on Intelligent Computing and Communication for Smart World (I2C2SW)*, 2018; pp 131–135. DOI: 10.1109/I2C2SW45816.2018.8997153.
22. 22. Xu, X., Guan, Y., Li, J. et al. Automatic glaucoma detection based on transfer induced attention network. *BioMed Eng OnLine 20*, 39 (2021). https://doi.org/10.1186/s12938-021-00877-5

CHAPTER 10

Automated Segregation of Lymphoid and Myeloid Blasts in Acute Leukemia Cases Using a Deep Convolutional Neural Network

K. K. ANILKUMAR[1], V. J. MANOJ[1], and T. M. SAGI[2]

[1]*Department of Electronics & Communication, Cochin University College of Engineering Kuttanad, Cochin University of Science and Technology, Cochin, Kerala, India*

[2]*Department of Medical Laboratory Technology, St. Thomas College of Allied Health Sciences, Changanacherry, Kerala, India*

ABSTRACT

An abnormal rise in the count of immature white blood cells in the blood and bone marrow along with reduction in the count of normal blood cells may be an indication of leukemia. Classification of acute leukemia into lymphoblastic or myeloblastic is carried out by pathologists or hematopathologists based on the morphological differences of the blast cells and with the support of cytochemical stains. Image-processing methods using *machine learning* can be used to classify leukemia by analyzing and processing images of bone marrow or blood smears. Such methods are simple, fast, and easy and can be used for assisting *pathologists* for a speedy classification of leukemia into various types and subtypes. This study performs automated classification of acute leukemia by segregating single blast cells into lymphoblasts and myeloblasts using *ResNet50*, a pretrained

Applied Intelligence for Medical Image Analysis. Aarti, Raju Pal, Mukesh Saraswat, & Himanshu Mittal (Eds.)

residual *deep convolutional neural network*, without the involvement of any image segregation and hand-crafted feature extraction. The proposed work successfully classified acute leukemia cells into lymphoblasts and myeloblasts with a classification accuracy of 94.9% using the pretrained network ResNet50. This chapter established that preprocessing techniques such as filtering, image enrichment, image segregation, and feature extraction are not necessary for the classification of leukemia smear images by *deep learning* methods. Classification of acute leukemia alone is considered in the study and classification of other types of leukemia can be done in future works.

10.1 INTRODUCTION

Leukemia is a malignant neoplasm of the blood-forming organs of the body including bone marrow and the lymphatic system.[1,2] In leukemia, an unusual spread of immature white blood cells (WBCs) known as *blasts* leads to a significant drop in the number of other normal blood cells. The human blood has three types of cells: Erythrocytes or red blood cells, leukocytes or WBCs, and thrombocytes or platelets.[1] Leukocytes are further classified into neutrophils (40–70%), lymphocytes (20–40%), monocytes (2–10%), eosinophils (1–6%), and basophils (<1%). Leukemia can be called a cancer of leukocytes and occurs in various forms which differ in their clinical, pathological, and hematological features.[2] According to the clinical course, leukemia is classified as *acute* and *chronic*, and based on the cell line mostly involved in the leukemic process, it is classified as *lymphoid* and *myeloid*.[1,2] This leads to four main categories of leukemia: *acute myeloid leukemia (AML), chronic myeloid leukemia, acute lymphoblastic leukemia (ALL), and chronic lymphocytic leukemia.* Acute leukemia generally follows an aggressive clinical course which, if left untreated, rapidly results in death in majority of patients.[2] On the other hand, in the case of chronic leukemia, the progression of the disease is slow compared to acute leukemia.

According to the criteria prescribed by the World Health Organization, presence of 20% or more blasts in the bone marrow can be considered as an indication of acute leukemia and the classification into ALL and AML is done on the basis of the morphological differences and using cytochemistry, which is the study of chemical elements in the cytoplasm of the cells.[2] The size of *lymphoblast* is usually 2–3 times the size of lymphocyte, whereas the size of *myeloblast* is about 3–5 times that of the lymphocyte.[1] In lymphoblast, the cytoplasm is scanty and without granules, whereas in myeloblast, the cytoplasm is scanty to moderate and may have granules in it.[1] The nuclear chromatin is uniform and coarse in lymphoblast and with 1 or 2 nucleoli, while in myeloblast, the chromatin is uniform and fine with the presence of 3–5 prominent nucleoli.[1] Differentiating ALL and AML based on the morphological differences by manually analyzing the blood and bone marrow smear using microscope may be sometimes difficult due to their visual similarities and hence cytochemical stains need to be used for the classification.

Aus et al.[3] suggested that image-processing-based techniques can be used to detect leukemia-associated morphological features in blast cells and such automated methods can be used to support the *pathologists* for an easy and speedy diagnosis of the disease in the initial phase itself. Such methods are simple, cost-effective, and quick and do not bias by the skill and expertise of the professionals who carry out the diagnostic procedures. Moreover, the images can easily and quickly be transmitted over long distances for remote diagnosis by experts.[4] Ample research has already taken place in the field of computer-aided detection of leukemia and many scholars have used various methods and analysis to spot and classify leukemia.[5]

10.2 RELATED STUDIES

Previous works in the field of computer-aided detection and classification of leukemia, especially ALL and AML, along with the recent studies using deep learning (DL) in the associated area are briefed in Table 10.1. In the studies using DL alone for detection of leukemia, the maximum accuracy was achieved by the work in Jha and Dutta,[6] but they have used image segmentation by mutual information (MI)–related hybrid model before the classification phase. The study in Rehman et al.[7] detects leukemia using *convolutional neural network* (CNN) features and classification by support vector machine (SVM) and obtained an accuracy of 99.2%. The works[10,11] used *DL* for categorizing WBCs and the maximum accuracy among these is 96.1%. The studies[12–15] tried detection and classification of both ALL and AML using some image segregation, feature extraction, and classification by *artificial neural network* or *fuzzy* techniques and a maximum accuracy of 99.8% is the highest in this category. All the other works cited in the table

TABLE 10.1 Related Studies.

Authors	Application area	Segmentation method	Features used	Classifier	Dataset used	Accuracy (%)
Jha and Dutta[6]	ALL	MI[a]-based hybrid model	Statistical and LDP[b]	CNN[c], deep learning	ALL-IDB2	98.7
Amjad Rahman et al.[7]	ALL	Thresholding	CNN features	CNN, deep learning	Amreek Clinical Lab, Pakistan	97.78
Jakkrich Laosai et al.[8]	ALL and AML	*k*-Means	Color, shape, and texture	*k*-Means and SVM[d]	Ubonratchathani Cancer Hospital	99.67
			CD[e] Marker	Deep learning	Sunpasit International Hospital, Thailand	
Luis H. S. Vogado et al.[9]	Leukemia	Not used	CNN features	DL[f], SVM	ALL-IDB, Hybrid	99.2
A. I. Shahin et al.[10]	WBC classification	Not used	CNN features	CNN, deep learning	ALL-IDB	96.1
Feiwei Qin et al.[11]	WBC classification	Not used	CNN features	CNN, deep learning	Private dataset	76.84
Jyoti Rawat et al.[12]	ALL and AML	Otsu's thresholding	Geometry, color, and texture	SVM	ASH	99.5
Ahmed S. Negum et al.[13]	ALL and AML	*k*-Means	Color, shape, size, and texture	ANN[7], decision tree	ALL-IDB	99.517
Balacel N. et al.[14]	ALL and AML	Not used	Shape	Fuzzy	Cliniques Universitaires, Belgium	96.4
Madhloom et al.[15]	ALL and AML	Region growing	Shape, color, and texture	SRG[8] segmentation	Malaya Medical Center, ALL-IDB	99.8
Madhloom et al.[16]	ALL	Morphological reconstruction	Shape and texture	*k*-NN[9]	Malaya Medical Center, Malaysia	92

TABLE 10.1 *(Continued)*

Authors	Application area	Segmentation method	Features used	Classifier	Dataset used	Accuracy (%)
Fabio Scotti[17]	ALL	Otsu's thresholding	Shape	Bayes, *k*-NN, FFNN[10]	ALL-IDB	–
Lorenzo Putzu et al.[18]	ALL	Zack algorithm	Shape, color, and texture	SVM	ALL-IDB	>90
Jyoti Rawat et al.[19]	ALL	Otsu's thresholding	Shape, color, and texture	SVM	ALL-IDB	89.8
Nimesh Patel et al.[20]	ALL	Zack algorithm and *k*-means	Shape, color, and texture	SVM	ALL-IDB	93.57
Siew Chin Neoh et al.[21]	ALL	Watershed and SDM[11]	Shape, texture, and color	MLP[12], SVM, and ensemble	ALL-IDB	96.72
Hussam N. Fakhouri et al.[22]	Leukemia types	Thresholding	Shape	SVM	Various online image banks	–
J. Rodellar et al.[23]	Leukemia types	Watershed	Geometric, color, and texture	SVM	Images from 374 patients in Spain	90.3
Sos Agaian et al.[24]	AML	*k*-Means	HD[13], shape, texture, and color	SVM	ASH	98
Subrajeet Mohapatra et al.[25]	ALL	*k*-Means	HD, shape, and texture	SVM	Ispat General Hospital, India	95
Preetham Kumar et al.[26]	AML	*k*-Means	Shape and texture	SVM	ASH	95
MoradiAmin et al.[27]	ALL	FCM[14]	Geometric and texture	Ensemble SVM	Al-Zahra and Omid Hospital, Iran	96.5–98.85

[a]*Mutual information,* [b]*local direction pattern,* [c]*convolutional neural network,* [d]*support vector machine,* [e]*cluster designation,* [f]*deep learning,* [g]*artificial neural network,* [h]*seeded region growing,* [i]*k-nearest neighbor,* [j]*feed forward neural network,* [k]*stimulating discriminant measures,* [l]*multilayer perceptron,* [m]*Hausdorff dimension,* [n]*fuzzy C-means clustering.*

also used some methods for segmenting the image, feature extraction, and classification by some kind of *machine learning* (ML)–based techniques and obtained accuracies varying from 89.8% to 98.85%.

10.3 PROPOSED METHOD

The conventional method of an image classification problem attempted by most of the works found in the literature was to use *preprocessing*, *image segregation*, and *feature extraction* before the actual classification phase. All these techniques involve intense computations which are generally difficult to perform and may affect the natural quality of the images. Moreover, such computationally exhaustive methods are difficult to follow by medical professionals for whom these methodologies are expected to help. On the other hand, DL-related methods are simple and they can classify images *without image segregation and hand-engineered feature extraction*, and the only preprocessing needed is to resize the images to match with the input image size of the DL network. The proposed method thus uses a simplified classification framework using DL which can be represented as shown in Figure 10.1, replacing the conventional classification framework.

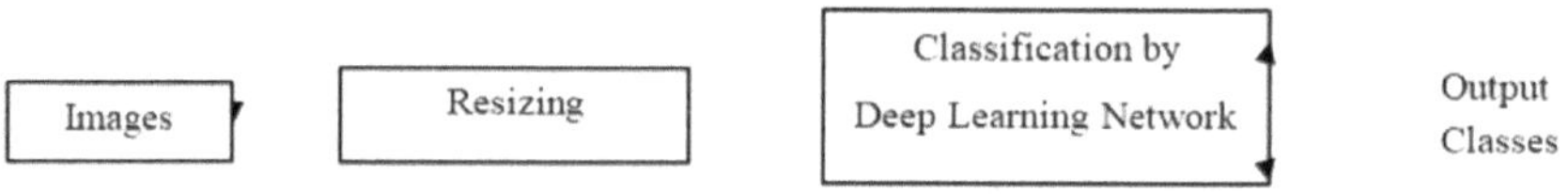

FIGURE 10.1 A simple classification framework using DL.

The main contributions of this study related to leukemia detection can be highlighted as follows: Automated detection of ALL and AML by segregating lymphoid and myeloid blast cells of acute leukemia smear images of a publicly available dataset using *ResNet50*, a pretrained residual deep convolutional neural network (DNN) without the involvement of image segmentation and feature extraction.

10.4 EXPERIMENTAL METHODS AND MATERIALS

The picture quality is not a big problem in DL-based classification,[28] and hence, the image classification setup based on DL is very simple unlike in classical image-processing and ML methods which need preprocessing, image segregation, and feature extraction blocks before the classification stage. Figure 10.2 shows the schematic setup of the classification scheme used in the proposed work. The dataset images are first cropped to get subimages which consist of single-cell images of the blasts, and these single-cell images are then resized to match with the image input size of the deep CNN. The features required for classifying the images are learned automatically by the CNN and the fully connected (FC) layer maps these features to one of the output classes. All classification experiments in this work were carried out using MATLAB 2019b in a computer with Intel Core i5 7th generation CPU @ 2.5GHz with 12 GB RAM.

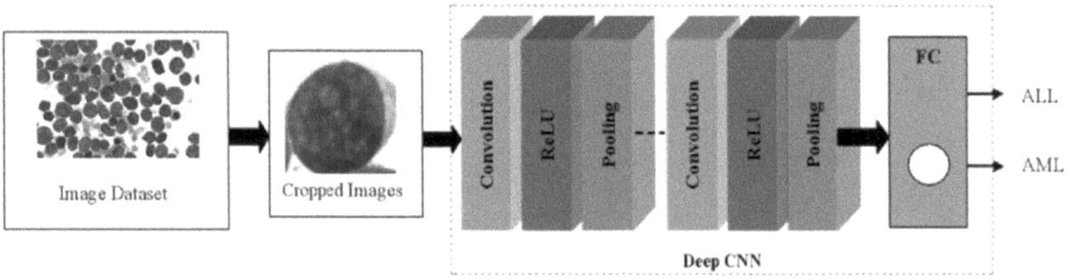

FIGURE 10.2 Block scheme of classification setup.

10.4.1 IMAGE DATASET

The images used in the proposed work were collected from an online image bank of the American Society of Hematology (ASH)[29] which consists of good-quality images of various pathological disorders including leukemia. We downloaded 80 smear images of ALL and 100 images of AML which consists of all subtypes of ALL and AML; 487 single lymphoblast cell images and another 487 myeloblast cell images are then manually cropped from the whole smear images of ASH image bank and these cropped images are then used as the dataset for the classification. Figure 10.3 shows sample downloaded images of ALL and AML and its cropped single blast cell versions.

10.4.2 CONVOLUTIONAL NEURAL NETWORKS

Even though CNNs vary in architecture and the number of layers used, most of the DL networks consist of the layers depicted in Figure 10.4.[30,31]

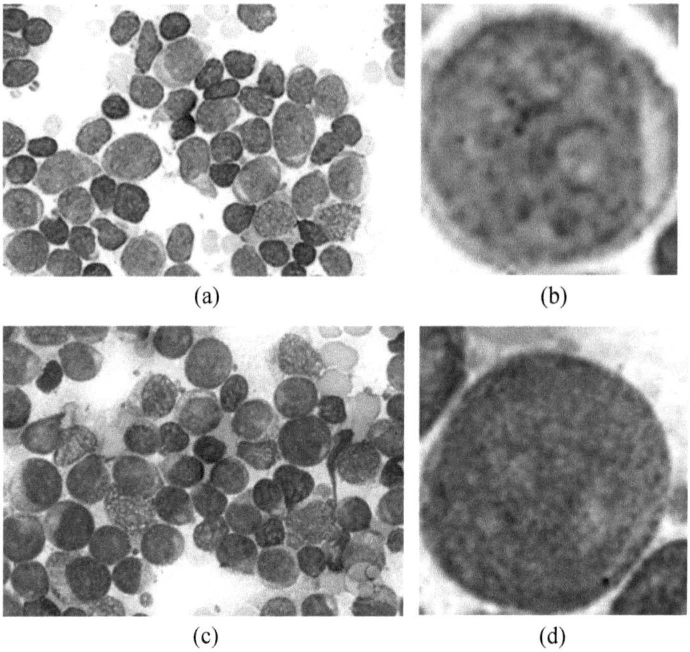

FIGURE 10.3 Sample images of ALL and AML: (a) ALL, (b) lymphoblast, (c) AML, and (d) myeloblast.

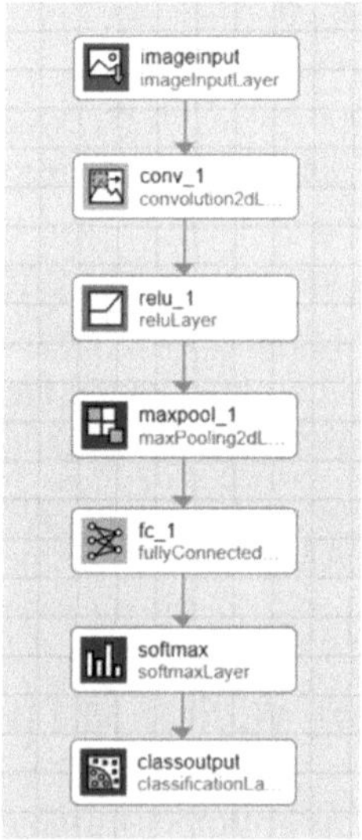

FIGURE 10.4 General architecture of a CNN.

CNNs are widely used in DL and they are highly suitable for images when given as inputs. CNNs are enthused from biological arrangements of a visual cortex which consists of simple and complex cells.[32] These cells stimulate based on subregions of the visual fields known as receptive fields. Similarly, the neurons of a convolutional layer are connected to the subregions of the previous layer rather than being FC as in classical neural networks. Hence, these neurons are not responsive for areas outside the subregions in the image.

10.4.3 PRETRAINED NETWORKS AND TRANSFER LEARNING

There are several pretrained DL networks available which are trained on greater than a million of general images like pen, pencil, keyboard, mouse, cup, birds, and animals, and many of these networks can classify images into 1000 mutually exclusive classes.[33] The proposed work uses *ResNet50*,[34,36] a pretrained residual deep CNN for the classification task. ResNet50 is a pretrained residual CNN which has a depth of 50 and trained on greater than a million of commonly available images. The CNN has an input image size of 224 × 224 and there are 177 layers. But such pretrained CNNs cannot be directly used to classify new images, such as leukemia smear images, because the networks are not trained on such datasets. The pretrained networks need to be adapted and trained on the new dataset before using it for classification of new images. The method of adapting a pretrained CNN to train on a new dataset to learn its new features is called *transfer learning*.[34] Adapting and fine-tuning a CNN to capture the features of a new dataset is easy compared to designing and training a new CNN fresh from the beginning. The parameters of the last learnable layers of ResNet50 are adjusted to match with our leukemia dataset and the size of all images is modified to suit the input image size of ResNet50 before the training is initiated.

10.4.4 DATA AUGMENTATION

The classification accuracy of a DL network is usually high when the dataset is very large. An augmented image data store can be used to modify the size of the images automatically and additional data augmentation techniques like flipping the images in the training set randomly along the vertical axis, translating the images few pixels vertically and horizontally, rotation, scaling, and so on can be applied to prevent the CNN from overfitting.[35] The proposed study also used such data augmentation techniques to manage network overfitting.

10.4.5 TRAINING ALGORITHM

During the training of CNN, the parameters of the network (weights and biases) are updated based on the training algorithm to minimize the loss function. This study used the training algorithm Adaptive Moment estimation (ADAM)[30,37] while carrying out training with the images in the dataset.

10.4.6 EVALUATION MATRICES

To compare the performance of different classification experiments, we used the parameters *accuracy*, *sensitivity*, *specificity*, *positive predictive value*, and *negative predictive value*, listed below, which are generally used in ML-related classification works. These evaluation parameters are computed by plotting the confusion matrices.[38]

$$Accuracy = \frac{TP + TN}{TP + TN + FP + FN}$$

$$Sensitivity = \frac{TP}{TP + FN}$$

$$Specificity = \frac{TN}{TN + FP}$$

$$Positive\ predictive\ value\ (PPV) = \frac{TP}{TP + FP}$$

$$Negative\ predictive\ value\ (NPV) = \frac{TN}{TN + FN}$$

where TP means true positive, TN means true negative, FP means false positive, and FN means false negative.

10.5 RESULTS AND DISCUSSION

The pretrained network, *ResNet50*, is trained by performing transfer learning and using ADAM algorithm on the cropped leukemia image dataset of ASH in such a way that 70% of images are randomly allotted for training. The remaining 20% images are used for validation and 10% for testing so that these images are not used for training. A validation accuracy of 94.33% is achieved in segregating the lymphoblasts and myeloblasts of acute leukemia cases. We have used an initial learning rate of 0.00006, 10 epochs, and validation frequency of 5. Learning rate schedule is also used to drop the learning rate by 50% after completing 5 epochs. A total training time of 176 min and 51 s has taken in a single CPU-based computer system. *A classification accuracy of 94.9% is achieved in the testing phase* and Figure 10.5 shows few classification images with the associated probabilities of residing to that class. The evaluation parameters of the classification are then calculated using the confusion matrix and the results are summarized in Table 10.2.

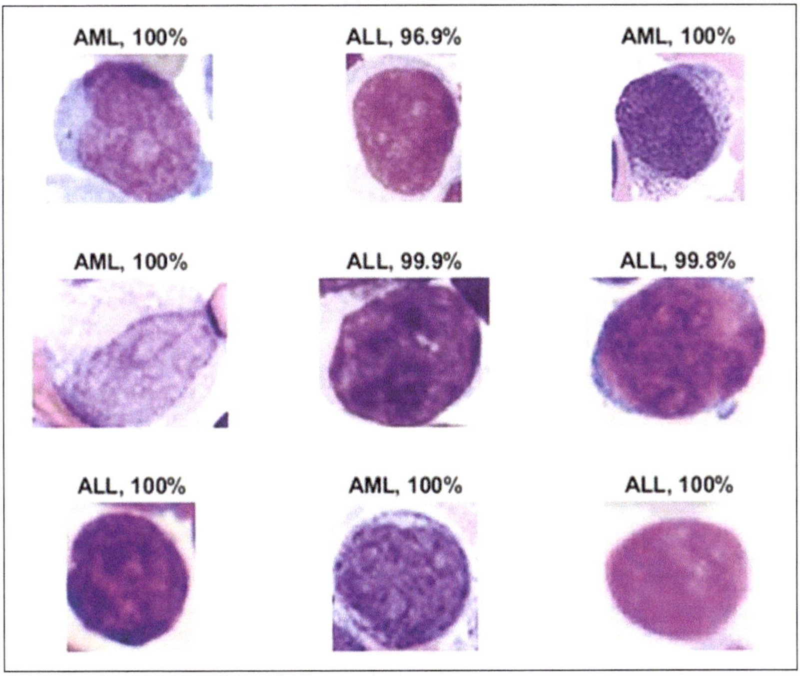

FIGURE 10.5 Sample classification images and associated probabilities with ResNet50.

TABLE 10.2 Confusion Matrix and Evaluation Parameters of ResNet50.

Confusion matrix		Predicted class		Accuracy (%)	Sensitivity (%)	Specificity (%)	PPV (%)	NPV (%)
		ALL	AML					
True class	ALL	47	2	94.9	95.92	93.88	94	95.83
	AML	3	46	94.9	93.88	95.92	95.83	94

The overall accuracy of 94.9% is obtained in classifying the blast cell images into ALL and AML by processing the data in its raw form, without involving any image enhancement technique, image segmentation, and feature extraction. It can be seen from Figure 10.5 that many images are classified with 100% probability of residing to that particular class. Forty-seven ALL blasts out of 49 images in the testing phase are correctly classified and 46 out of 49 AML images are also correctly classified. The sensitivity, which is the ability of the classifier in identifying the positive cases, is slightly better for ALL cases compared to that of the AML cases. The classification time of 176 min and 51 s can be attributed to the fact that ResNet50 is a residual DL network having a depth of 50 with a total of 177 layers. The classification time can be reduced to a good extent by means of computers with graphics processing unit to support parallel processing.

A comparison of the performance of this study with other related works is shown in Table 10.3. Classification using DL alone is carried out in works Jha and Dutta[6] and Rehman et al.[7] and obtained an accuracy of 98.7% and 97.74%, respectively; but they have used image segmentation before the classification phase. Laosai et al.[8] used both DL and SVM for classifying ALL and AML and also used image segmentation for obtaining a maximum accuracy of 99.67% and the accuracy in segregating lymphoid and myeloid blasts was 98.62% using DL. Vogado et al.[9] have done the detection of leukemia without using any image segmentation, like the proposed work, but they have used DL and SVM together for classification and obtained an accuracy of 99.2% for the general detection of leukemia. In the proposed work, using pretrained network ResNet50, an accuracy of 94.9% is achieved using DL alone for classifying acute leukemia into ALL and AML. *No other works available in the literature used such a simple classification setup using DL alone and without image segregation and feature extraction, for classifying leukemia images.* The classification accuracy is slightly less because DNNs need large dataset to produce excellent results and our leukemia image dataset, with 487 images

TABLE 10.3 Performance Comparison with Related Works.

Authors	Application	Segmentation	Classifier	Dataset (%)	Accuracy
Jha and Dutta[6]	ALL	MI based	DNN	ALL_IDB2	98.7
Rehman et al.[7]	ALL	Thresholding	DNN	Private dataset	97.74
Laosai et al.[8]	ALL and AML	*k*-Means	DNN, SVM	Private dataset	99.67
Vogado et al.[9]	Leukemia	Not used	DNN, SVM	ALL-IDB, hybrid	99.2
Rawat et al.[12]	ALL and AML	Otsu's threshold	SVM	ASH	99.5
Negum et al.[13]	ALL and AML	*k*-Means	ANN	ALL-IDB	99.52
Balacel N. et al.[14]	ALL and AML	Not used	Fuzzy	Private	96.4
Madhloom et al.[18]	ALL and AML	Region growing	SRG	Private and ALL-IDB	99.8
Proposed method	**ALL and AML**	**Not used**	**DNN**	**ASH**	**94.9**

in each class, was not so large. Balacel et al.[14] performed classification of ALL and AML without image segmentation and obtained an accuracy of 96.4% using fuzzy classifier on a private dataset. Other related works[12,13,15] also used some technique of image segmentation before the classification phase to detect ALL and AML.

10.6 CONCLUSION

Quick diagnosis of the acute leukemia is very important as the progression of the disease is very fast and automated detection systems can be used to support the *Pathologists* for a speedy and easy diagnosis. DL is a new branch of ML and only a very few studies available in the literature related to automated detection systems for leukemia using DL. The proposed work outlined the use of DL network for automated classification of leukemia into ALL and AML using a dataset of ASH which is publicly available. The most protruding feature of the study is that all the classifications carried out by the deep CNN were performed without the use of any image segmentation and hand-engineered feature extraction techniques that involve intense computations. The present work managed to classify the acute leukemia images of ASH dataset into ALL and AML with 94.9% accuracy with a pretrained residual DL network ResNet50. Classification of leukemia images into ALL and AML alone is attempted in the study and further research can be initiated by investigating with other types of leukemia images so that classification of leukemia smear images into other types and subtypes can be done.

ACKNOWLEDGMENTS

The authors are grateful to the American Society of Hematology (ASH) for providing good-quality image datasets of leukemia.

CONFLICT OF INTEREST

The authors do not have any conflicts of interest to declare in connection with the publication of this manuscript.

KEYWORDS

- **acute leukemia**
- **microscopic smear images**
- **lymphoid cells**
- **myeloid cells**
- **deep learning**
- **convolutional neural networks**
- **pretrained networks**
- **transfer learning**

REFERENCES

1. Henry, J. B. *Clinical Diagnosis and Management by Laboratory Methods*, 17th ed.; WB Saunders Company: Philadelphia, 1989.
2. Firkin, F.; Chesterman, C.; Penington, D.; Rush, B. *De Gruchy's Clinical Haematology in Medical Practice*, 5th ed.; Blackwell Publishing Sciences Ltd.: Oxford, UK, 1989.
3. Aus, H. M.; Harms, H.; Haucke, M.; Beritova, J.; ter Meulen, V.; Gunzer, U.; Baumann, I.; Abmayr, W. Leukaemia-Related Morphological Features in Blast Cells. *Cytometry* **1986,** *7* (4), 365–370. DOI: 10.1002/cyto.990070411.
4. Anilkumar, K. K.; Manoj, V. J.; Sagi, T. M. Colour Based Image Segmentation for Automated Detection of Leukaemia: A Comparison between CIELAB and CMYK Colour Spaces. In *Proceedings of the IEEE International Conference Circuits and Systems in Digital Enterprise Technology*; 2018; pp 1–6. DOI: 10.1109/ICCSDET.2018.8821067.
5. Alsalem, M. A.; Zaidan, A. A.; Zaidan, B. B.; Hashim, M.; Madhloom, H. T.; Azeez, N. D. A Review of Automatic Detection and Classification of Acute Leukemia: Coherent Taxonomy, Datasets, Validation and Performance Measurements, Motivation, Open Challenges and Recommendations. *Comput. Method Prog. Biol.* **2018,** *158*, 93–112.
6. Jha, K.; Dutta, H. S. Mutual Information Based Hybrid Model and Deep Learning for Acute Lymphoblastic Leukemia Detection in Single Cell Blood Smear Images. *Comput. Method Prog. Biol.* **2019,** *179*, 1–12.
7. Rehman, A.; Abbas, N.; Saba, T.; Rahman, S. I. U.; Mehmood, Z.; Kolivand, H. Classification of Acute Lymphoblastic Leukemia Using Deep Learning. *Microsc. Res. Tech.* **2018,** *81* (11), 1310–1317. DOI: 10.1002/jemt.23139.
8. Laosai, J.; Chamnongthai, K. Classification of Acute Leukemia Using Medical-Knowledge-Based Morphology and CD Marker. *Biomed. Signal Process.* **2018,** *44*, 127–137.

9. Vogado, L. H. S.; Veras, R. M. S.; Araujo, F. H. D.; Silva, R. R. V.; Aires, K. R. T. Leukemia Diagnosis in Blood Slides Using Transfer Learning in CNNs and SVM for Classification. *Eng. Appl. Artif. Intell.* **2018,** *72*, 415–422. DOI: 10.1016/j.engappai. 2018.04.024.
10. Shahin, A. I.; Guo, Y.; Amin, K. M.; Sharawi, A. A. White Blood-Cell Identification System Based on Convolutional Deep Neural Learning Networks. *Comput. Methods Programs Biomed.* **2019,** *168*, 69–80. DOI: 10.1016/j.cmpb.2017.11.015.
11. Qin, Feiwei; Gao, N.; Peng, Y.; Wu, Zizhao; Shen, S. Artur Grudtsin; Fine-Grained Leukocyte Classification with Deep Residual Learning for Microscopic Images. *Comput. Method Prog. Biol.* **2018,** *162*, 243–252.
12. Rawat, J.; Singh, A.; Hs, B.; Virmani, J.; Devgun, J. S. Computer Assisted Classification Framework for Prediction of Acute Lymphoblastic Acute Myeloblastic Leukemia. *Biocybern. Biomed. Eng.* **2017,** *37* (4), 637–654. DOI: 10.1016/j.bbe.2017.07.003.
13. Ahmed, S. Negum; Osama A. Hassam; Ahmed H. Kandil; A Decision Support System for Acute Leukemia Classification Based on Digital Microscopic Images. *Alex. Eng. J.* **2018,** *57* (4), 2319–2332.
14. Belacel, N.; Vincke, P.; Scheiff, J. M.; Boulassel, M. R. Acute Leukemia Diagnosis Aid Using Multicriteria Fuzzy Assignment Methodology. *Comput. Methods Programs Biomed.* **2001,** *64* (2), 145–151. DOI: 10.1016/s0169-2607(00)00100-0.
15. Madhloom, H. T.; Kareem, S. A.; Ariffin, H. Computer Aided Acute Leukemiia Blast Cell Segmentation in Peripheral Blood Images. *J. Vibroeng.* **2015,** *17* (8), 4517–4532.
16. Madhloom, H. T.; Kareem, S. A.; Ariffin, H. A Robust Feature Extraction and Selection Method for the Recognition of Lyphocytes versus Acute Lymphoblastic Leukemia. In *Proceedings of the International Conference Advanced Computer Science Applications and Technologies*; 2012. DOI: 10.1109/ACSAT.2012.62.
17. Scotti, F. Automatic Morphological Analysis for Acute Leukemia Identification in Peripheral Blood Microscopic Images. In *Proceedings of the IEEE International Conference Computational Intelligence for Measurement Systems and Applications*; 2005; pp 96–101. DOI: 10.1109/CIMSA.2005.1522835.
18. Putzu, L.; Caocci, G.; Di Ruberto, C. Leukocyte Classification for Leukemia Detection Using Image Processing Techniques. *Artif. Intell. Med.* **2014,** *62* (3), 179–191. DOI: 10.1016/j.artmed.2014.09.002.
19. Rawat, J.; Singh, A.; Bhadauria, H. S.; Virmani, J.; Devgun, J. S. Classification of Acute Lymphoblastic Leukemia Using Hybrid Hierarchical Classifiers. *Multimed. Tools Appl.* **2017,** *76* (18), 19057–19085. DOI: 10.1007/s11042-017-4478-3.
20. Patel, N.; Mishra, A. Automated Leukemia Detection Using Microscopic Images. *Proc. Second Int. Symp. Comput. Vision Internet Proc. Comput. Sci.* **2015,** *58*, 635–642. DOI: 10.1016/j.procs.2015.08.082
21. Neoh, S. C.; Srisukkham, W.; Zhang, L.; et al. An Intelligent Decision Support System for Leukaemia Diagnosis Using Microscopic Blood Images. *Sci. Rep.—UK* **2015,** *5*, 14938.
22. Begum, A. R. J.; Razak, T. A. Diagnosing Leukemia from Microscopic Images Using Image Analysis and Processing Techniques. In *Proceedings of the World Congress on Computing and Communication Technologies*; 2017; pp 227–230. DOI: 10.1109/WCCCT.2016.63.
23. Fakhouri, H. N.; Al-Sharaeh, S. H. A Hybrid Methodology for Automation the Diagnosis of Leukemia Based on Quantitative and Morphological Feature Analysis. *Mod. Appl. Sci.* **2018,** *12* (3), 56–73. DOI: 10.5539/mas.v12n3p56.

24. Rodellar, J.; Alférez, S.; Acevedo, A.; Molina, A.; Merino, A. Image Processing and Machine Learning in the Morphological Analysis of Blood Cells. *Int. J. Lab. Hematol.* **2018,** *40* (Suppl. 1), 46–53. DOI: 10.1111/ijlh.12818.
25. Mohapatra, S.; Patra, D.; Satpathy, S. Unsupervised Blood Microscopic Image Segmentation and Leukemia Detection Using Color Based Clustering. *Int. J. Comput. Inf. Syst. Ind. Manage. Appl.* **2012,** *4*, 477–485.
26. Kumar, P.; Udwadia, S. M. Automatic Detection of Acute Myeloid Leukemia for Microscopic Blood Smear Image. In *Proceedings of the International Conference Advanced Communications and Informatics*; 2017; pp 1803–1807. DOI: 10.1109/ICACCI.2017.8126106.
27. Moradi Amin, M.; Memari, A.; Samadzadehaghdam, N.; Kermani, S.; Talebi, A. Computer Aided Detection and Classification of Acute Lymphoblastic Leukemia Cell Subtypes Based on Microscopic Image Analysis. *Micro Sci. Res. Tech.* **2016,** *79*, 908–916.
28. Dodge, S.; Karam, L. Understanding How the Image Quality Affects Deep Neural Networks. In *Proceedings of the Eight IEE International Conference Quality of Multimedia Experience (QoMEX)*; 2016; pp 1–6. DOI: 10.1109/QoMEX.2016.7498955.
29. ASH Image Bank. http://imagebank.hematology.org/ (accessed December 4, 2019); American Society of Hematology.
30. Lecun, Y.; Bottou, L.; Bengio, Y.; Haffner, P. Gradient-Based Learning Applied to Document Recognition. *Proc. IEE* **1998,** *86* (11), 2278–2324. DOI: 10.1109/5.726791.
31. Szegedy, C.; Liu, W.; Jia, Y.; Sermanet, P.; Reed, S.; Anguelov, D.; Erhan, D.; Vanhoucke, V.; Rabinovich, A. Going Deeper with Convolutions. In *Proceedings of the IEEE Conference on Computer Vision and Pattern Recognition (CVPR)*; 2015; pp 1–9. DOI: 10.1109/CVPR.2015.7298594.
32. Hubel, D. H.; Wiesel, T. N. Receptive Fields of Single Neurones in the Cat's Striate Cortex. *J. Physiol.* **1959,** *148* (3), 574–591. DOI: 10.1113/jphysiol.1959.sp006308.
33. Russakovsky, O.; Deng, J.; Su, H.; Krause, J.; Satheesh, S.; Ma, S.; Huang, Z.; Karpathy, A.; Khosla, A.; Bernstein, M.; Berg, A. C.; Fei-Fei, L. ImageNet Large Scale Visual Recognition Challenge. *Int. J. Comput. Vis.* **2015,** *115* (3), 211–252. DOI: 10.1007/s11263-015-0816-y.
34. He, K.; Zhang, X.; Ren, S.; Sun, J. Deep Residual Learning for Image Recognition. In *Proceedings of the IEEE Conference on Computer Vision and Pattern Recognition*; 2016; pp 770–778. DOI: 10.1109/CVPR.2016.90.
35. Anilkumar, K. K.; Manoj, V. J.; Sagi, T. M. Automated Detection of Leukemia by Pretrained Deep Neural Networks and Transfer Learning: A Comparison. *Med. Eng. Phys.* **2021,** *98*, 8–19. DOI: 10.1016/j.medengphy.2021.10.006.
36. Srivastava, N.; Hinton, G.; Krizhevsky, A.; Sutskever, I.; Salakhutdinov, R. Dropout: A Simple Way to Prevent Neural Networks from Overfitting. *J. Mach. Learn. Res.* **2014,** *15*, 1929–1958.
37. Kingma, D.; Ba, J. *Adam: A Method for Stochastic Optimization, arXiv* **2014**. p 1412.6980. Preprint arXiv.
38. Anilkumar, K. K.; Manoj, V. J.; Sagi, T. M. Automated Detection of B Cell and T Cell Acute Lymphoblastic Leukaemia Using Deep Learning. *IRBM* **2022,** *43* (5), 405–413. DOI: 10.1016/j.irbm.2021.05.005.

CHAPTER 11

Evaluation of Deep Learning Network Architectures for Medicine Expenditure Prediction in the Healthcare Domain

ULISES MANUEL RAMIREZ-ALCOCER[1],
JACIEL DAVID HERNANDEZ-RESENDIZ[1], and EDGAR TELLO LEAL[2]

[1]*Multidisciplinary Academic Unit Reynosa-Rodhe, Autonomous University of Tamaulipas, Reynosa, Tamaulipas, Mexico*

[2]*Faculty of Engineering and Science, Autonomous University of Tamaulipas, Victoria, Tamaulipas, Mexico*

In this chapter, we present the evaluation of four architectures based on deep learning (DL): long short-term memory (LSTM), stacked LSTM, convolutional neural network (CNN)-LSTM, and Encoder-Decoder LSTM. These architectures are implemented to predict drug expenditures over time that patients may incur when permanently prescribed a medication. We propose a methodology to select the inference model that achieves the best performance in the training stage of the DL network in each architecture. The experiment uses a healthcare dataset consisting of records of patient orders to provide a group of analgesics for 1565 days. When evaluating DL-based models, the metrics of root mean square error (RMSE), root mean square error (RMSLE), mean absolute error (MAE), and mean absolute percentage error (MAPE) are used, highlighting the models of CNN-LSTM and encoder-decoder LSTM, which obtain the best performance in the implemented experimentation.

Applied Intelligence for Medical Image Analysis. Aarti, Raju Pal, Mukesh Saraswat, & Himanshu Mittal (Eds.)

11.1 INTRODUCTION

Health care is a constantly growing area, and in some countries, it is a booming economic sector. In health care, there are significant challenges related to operating costs and patient care (health-care service), quality of service, and the complexity of organizational processes,[1] the incorporation of information technologies, and data analysis to improve the accuracy of health-care-related activities.[2]

Health-care institutions are adopting information technology-based approaches to support management models (internal operation or external operation),[3] including support for patient care, diagnosis, medical treatment, patient discharge, and postdischarge follow-up care of the patient.[4] Management systems for external collaboration refer to the relationship with providers, as well as with patients. Most of the advances in automation through information technology in health processes are focused on patients. Automating the processes has made possible the generation and collection of large amounts of information through these information systems.[5]

Data-driven decision-making can collaborate to address the challenges of the health-care domain,[6] facilitating the transition to a health-care industry built on the value of data. In this sense, data analytics derived from data mining, machine learning, or deep learning (DL) provides techniques to extract information from complex processes and big data for processing and analysis to support decision-making in health care.[7,8]

In this way, predicting the health-care expenditure that patients diagnosed with a critical illness face is a requirement of great importance in data analytics in health care. Further, the prediction of health-care spending is of interest to government health-care assistance services, hospitals, health insurance companies, drug manufacturers, and distributors.[9] The main problem focuses on constructing inference models with high precision and performance in predicting future drug and service spending, allowing patients to plan to spend in the short, medium, and long term, choosing an appropriate insurance plan. Similarly, health-care institutions can define better cost planning from a business viewpoint.

The DL techniques have demonstrated their ability to improve the discriminative power compared with other machine learning methods. Recurrent neural networks (RNN) are DL techniques inspired by the human nervous system and the brain's structure to find optimal solutions to complex problems through an internal structure of layers, blocks, and neurons. RNN can solve different problems, including dimensionality reduction, pattern recognition, classification, clustering, regression, and predictive analysis.[10] The long short-term memory (LSTM) is a DL technique that is seen as the most efficient method of time series prediction, and the convolutional neural network (CNN) obtains excellent values in the evaluation metrics in computer vision and image recognition problems.[11] DL networks have been applied in the health-care domain, for example, in predicting health-care trajectories using historical patient care records,[12] predicting patient's spending on medications,[13] analyzing longitudinal patient records,[14] early diagnose of cardiovascular diseases from electrocardiograph,[15] and diagnosis of gastric lesions.[16]

In this chapter, we evaluate the performance of a set of DL neural network algorithms implemented to predict health-care spending. The deep network architectures implemented are LSTM, stacked LSTM, CNN-LSTM, and encoder-decoder LSTM. The performance of selected DL-based inference models is evaluated using root-mean-square error (RMSE), the root-mean-square-logarithmic error (RMSLE), the mean absolute error (MAE), and the mean absolute percentage error (MAPE) metrics. In addition, we propose a methodology to guide the selection of the best inference model, defining the data preprocessing of the input data to the neural network, design, training, and testing of the network model, and selection of the prediction model with the best performance. In the training and testing stages of the prediction models, the Truven MarketScan dataset is used, which consists of the multivariate time series type, which contains values of the purchase of pain medications most used in the USA. The results achieved by the inference models exceed state-of-the-art with similar approaches.

11.2 RELATED WORK

Recently, attempts have been made to use DL neural networks in the health-care domain for predicting medication expenditure. Next, the researches that are close to the proposed approach are described. In Zeng et al.,[17] a DL-based multiview framework is proposed to predict drug spending per client using historical data of claims submitted to insurance companies. In the approach, heterogeneous information is used, considering demographic characteristics, medical codes, use of drugs, and use of facilities. The dataset used was derived from pediatric information, containing approximately 8.5 million records of health-care information from around 450 thousand patients, which corresponds to a period of 24 months. The neural network is composed of the first view of a demographic encoder, in which the features are integrated into the vector representation through a forward neural network. In the second view, a utilization vector is generated, in which information on a patient's visits to the different areas of a hospital is represented. The usage encoder is built using a bi-LSTM network that captures the dependency between facility usage sequences. In a third view, the clinical information of the patient's visits to the doctor is cataloged through a scheme of medical codes, making it possible to build a medical encoder through a bidirectional neural network. In the last stage, the vectors corresponding to each view are concatenated to predict medical expenditure.

In Kaushik et al.,[18] a generative adversarial network model (GAN based on variance) is presented, allowing to reduce the variance difference between generated and the real data during the model training phase, using a dataset from the drug expenses for USA patients. The V-GAN model uses an LSTM network as a generating model and a CNN as a discriminatory model. The model proposed was compared to other GAN variants and machine learning approaches, surpassing the performance values of the reference prediction models. Similarly, in Kaushik et al.,[13] the prediction of drug expenditure using time series data, applying traditional and DL prediction methods, is discussed. The Auto-Regressive Integrated Moving Average (ARIMA), LSTM, and stacked LSTM are the methods implemented, using monthly drug spending data of more than 50,000 patients between 2011 and 2015, using 48 months for the training of the models and 12 months for the test stage. The stacked LSTM model obtains the best performance in the experimentation carried out.

In this sense, in Kaushik et al.,[19] the performance evaluation of different statistical techniques, neural networks, and a set of applications in predicting the average cost per week of pain medication costs is presented. The evaluated models are based on ARIMA, MLP, LSTM, and an assembly type model that combines the predictions of the ARIMA, MLP, and LSTM models. The results obtained reveal that the ensemble model performs better in predicting the consumption of pain medications. Moreover, in Kaushik et al.,[20] the implementation of multihead DL architectures

(LSTM, CNN-LSTM, and ConvLSTM) and the generation of an assembly model to predict the average expenditure on drugs in periods of 7 days are presented. The assembled model combines the predictions of the three multihead models using an exponential weight algorithm, outperforming the other models.

11.3 METHODOLOGY

11.3.1 FRAMEWORK

This section describes the proposed framework to select the inference model with the best performance, which comprises four stages: data preprocessing, network model design, training and testing of deep network models, and selection of the prediction model, as shown in Figure 11.1.

11.3.1.1 DATA PREPROCESSING

The objective of this stage is to prepare the input data for its correct interpretation by the prediction algorithms, which are composed of the following activities.

- **Data transformation to time-series:** This activity consists of forming a dataset in a time series format, assigning a window of seven instances to represent the purchases of medicines in 1 week.
- **Weekly average:** It consists of constructing a time series covering 1 week's data, having a single value per week calculating the average from the values contained in the period.
- **Data normalization:** In the values of the attributes of the dataset, a normalization of the min/max type is applied, allowing the characteristics to be transformed by scaling each characteristic to a specific range, making it possible to reduce the redundancy of the data.

11.3.1.2 NETWORK MODEL DESIGN

The stage consists of selecting the DL architectures that will be applied to predict costs in the hospital environment. In this stage, the following activities are carried out:

- **Select DL architecture:** The activity determines the architectures available on the platform, which enables the following activity.
- **Parameter capture:** In this activity, the operating parameters of each previously selected DL architecture are defined.

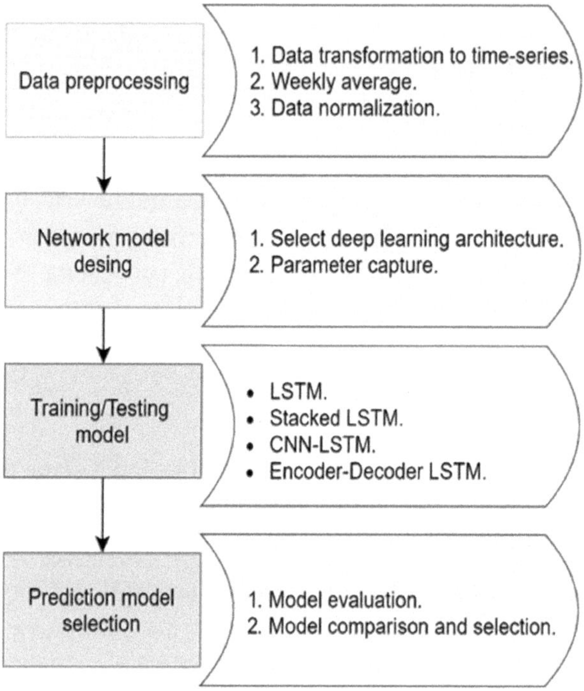

FIGURE 11.1 View of the stages and activities that form the methodology.

11.3.1.3 TRAINING/TESTING MODEL

At this stage, the selected DL architectures are trained and tested using the dataset processed in the first stage of the methodology (in this experimentation, LSTM, Stacked LSTM, CNN-LSTM, and encoder–decoder LSTM are implemented). The dataset is divided into a subdataset with 80% of the instances for the training stage. With the remaining 20% instances, a second subdataset is generated that will be employed for the testing stage. The subdatasets generated in this stage will be used to train and test the four selected architectures.

11.3.1.4 PREDICTION MODEL SELECTION

This stage consists of identifying and selecting the model with the best performance from calculating the error metrics, considering that this stage will be executed for each architecture of the selected deep network.

- **Model evaluation:** The performance of each model in the test phase is calculated using the RMSE (Eq. (11.1)), RMSLE (Eq. (11.2)), MAE (Eq. (11.3)), and MAPE (Eq. (11.4)) metrics.
- **Model comparison and selection:** A performance comparison is executed from the value obtained in the RMSE metric selected by the model with the lowest value in the metric.

Finally, Table 11.1 shows all the parameters defined in each of the DL architectures used in our experiment. These parameters allow the construction of each of the prediction models that generated the results described in the next section.

Figures 11.2 and 11.3 show the architectures of the DL CNN-LSTM and encoder–decoder LSTM networks. In these architectures, the parameters displayed in Table 11.1 were specified. In the DL architecture (see Figure 11.2), we design a model with one CNN layer, one max pooling layer, one LSTM layer, one dropout layer, and two dense layers with different parameters (see Table 11.1). The CNN-LSTM model is connected in a recurrent network to combine the advantages of a single LSTM layer with one CNN layer, making the model capable of learning higher-level temporal representations; furthermore, automatically extracting and learning features from one-dimensional sequence data. The first CNN layer interprets subsequences from the inputs (input vector), provided as a sequence to an LSTM model to interpret them as input and process them. That is, calculate the memory for the subsequent LSTM blocks. The network is trained for 100 epochs, a batch size of 64, and an optimizer Adamax is used.

On the other hand, in the DL architecture shown in Figure 11.3, the designed encoder–decoder model is presented. This model comprises two submodels: the encoder and the decoder. The encoder submodel uses an LSTM network with 200 units and ReLU-type activation. This submodel aims to read and interpret the input sequences, generating an output vector (fixed-length vector) that represents the interpretation of the input sequences obtained by the model. Subsequently, from a repeat

TABLE 11.1 Parameters of the DL Neural Networks.

Model	Hyperparameters	Value
LSTM	LSTM1 units	50
	LSTM1 activation	Relu
	Dense units	1
Stacked LSTM	LSTM1 units	100
	LSTM1 activation	Relu
	LSTM1 Return_sequences	True
	Dropout	0.1
	LSTM2 units	100
	LSTM2 activation	Relu
	LSTM2 Return_sequences	False
	Dense units	1
CNN-LSTM	Conv1D filters	64
	Conv1D padding	Same
	Conv1D Kernel_size	32
	Conv1D activation	Relu
	MaxPooling1D Pool_size	1
	LSTM1 units	100
	LSTM1 activation	Relu
	LSMT1 Return_sequences	True
	Dropout	0.2
	Dense1 units	100
	Dense1 activation	Relu
	Dense2 units	1
Encoder–decoder LSTM	LSTM1 units	200
	LSTM1 activation	Relu
	LSTM1 Return_sequences	False
	Dropout	0.1
	Repeat vector	1
	LSTM2 units	200
	LSTM2 activation	Relu
	LSTM2 Return_sequences	True
	TimeDistributed dense units	200
	TimeDistributed dense activation	Relu
	Dense units	1

vector-type layer, the output of the encoder submodel is repeated once for each time step required in the output sequence. This sequence is used by the decoder submodel, an LSTM layer with the same parameters as the LSTM encoder. The decoder submodel generates a value for each in the output time step, which a single output model can interpret. Subsequently, two output layers of the dense type are implemented, each layer within a TimeDistributed container, allowing the model output to be wrapped and thus using these output layers to make each prediction for each time step in the output sequence. The epochs, batch size and optimizer for training specified in this architecture are similar to those defined in the DL architecture above.

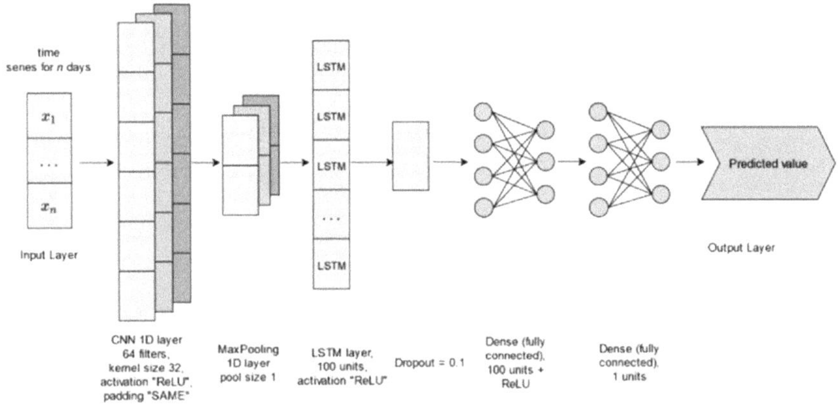

FIGURE 11.2 Architecture of CNN-LSTM model.

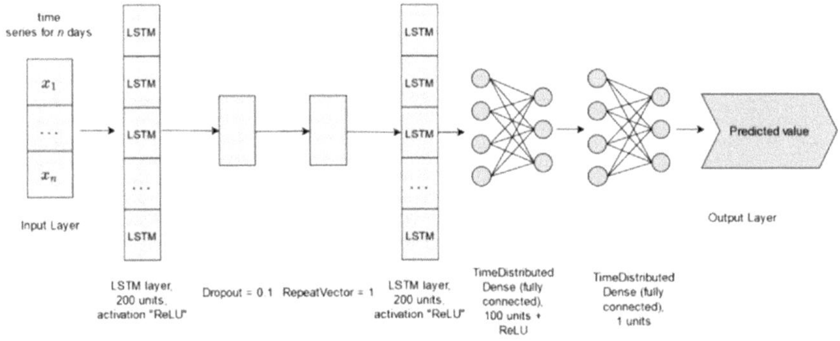

FIGURE 11.3 Architecture of encoder–decoder LSTM model.

11.3.2 MEASUREMENT

To evaluate the performance of the proposed approach, we adopted four classic error indicators: the RMSE, the RMSLE, the MAE, and the MAPE.

RMSE is the square root of the average squared errors between the predicted and experimental values calculated by Equation 11.1. RMSE is always a positive value, and a value 0 indicates a perfect prediction.

$$\text{RMSE} = \sqrt{\frac{1}{N}\sum_{i=1}^{N}(y_i - \hat{y}_i)^2} \tag{11.1}$$

where y_i denotes the true value or target value, $\hat{y}_i$ denotes the predicted value, and N denotes the number of evaluation samples. This notation is similar in Eqs. (11.2–11.4).

RMSLE is the logarithmic value of the mean of the residuals. Prediction errors can occur in both areas with small outliers and areas with large outliers. RMSLE helps reduce its effect by assigning penalties to items with underestimated outliers rather than those with overestimated outliers. RMSLE is calculated using the following equation:

$$\text{RMSE} = \sqrt{\frac{1}{N}\sum_{i=1}^{N}(y_i - \hat{y}_i)^2}$$

$$\text{RMSLE} = \sqrt{\frac{1}{N}\sum_{i=1}^{N}(\text{loglog}(\hat{y}_i + 1) - \text{loglog}(y_i + 1))^2} \tag{11.2}$$

MAE is the absolute error average and reflects the error between the actual value (y) and the predicted value ($\hat{y}$). The smaller the MAE is, the higher the accuracy the prediction achieves. The formula is as follows:

$$\text{RMSE} = \sqrt{\frac{1}{N}\sum_{i=1}^{N}(y_i - \hat{y}_i)^2}$$

$$\text{RMSLE} = \sqrt{\frac{1}{N}\sum_{i=1}^{N}\left(\log\log(\hat{y}_i + 1) - \log\log(y_i + 1)\right)^2}$$

$$\text{MAE} = \frac{1}{N}\sum_{i=1}^{N}|y_i - \hat{y}_i| \tag{11.3}$$

MAPE represents the ratio between the error and the actual value, that is, the error is defined as the actual value minus the predicted value. The smaller the MAPE is, the closer the predicted value is to the true value (Eq. 11.4).

$$\text{RMSE} = \sqrt{\frac{1}{N}\sum_{i=1}^{N}\left(y_i - \hat{y}_i\right)^2}$$

$$\text{RMSLE} = \sqrt{\frac{1}{N}\sum_{i=1}^{N}\left(\log\log\left(\hat{y}_i + 1\right) - \log\log\left(y_i + 1\right)\right)^2}$$

$$\text{MAPE} = \frac{1}{N}\sum_{i=1}^{N}\frac{\left|y_i - \hat{y}_i\right|}{y_i} \tag{11.4}$$

11.4 RESULTS

11.4.1 DATASET

The dataset contains historical information (from January 2011 to April 2015) about pain medication orders derived from the popular Truven MarketScan database. This dataset contains real-world health-care data, providing information about the top 10 most prescribed pain reliever medications in the United States. In our experiment, the two most commonly used drugs were selected, which we called drugs A and B, allowing us to generate a univariate time series that contains the mean expenditures of patients on these drugs. In this sense, 1428 patients refilled drug A per day, and approximately 550 patients reordered drug B each day. The data corresponding to 1250 days (80%) and 315 days are used for each prediction model's training and testing stage, respectively.

11.4.2 DESCRIPTIVE ANALYSIS

Table 11.2 shows a descriptive statistical analysis of the records in each drug's dataset. The average expenditure made by patients for drug A was 503.72 ± 42.86 (USD), while the average cost for drug B was 214.23 ± 51.64 (USD). Figure 11.4 shows the behavior of medication A consumption through a time series. The *X*-axis represents a time window of 7 days (per week), and the *Y*-axis represents the average value (USD) of medication A paid by patients. This figure shows a constant variation in drug expenditure, with a high trend with a substantial increase between weeks 165 and 215. On the other hand, Figure 11.5 shows the behavior over time of the mean expenditure of medication B, with a constant incremental trend every week, starting with an average cost of 150 USD and ending at 245 USD, with a maximum peak of 338 USD.

TABLE 11.2 Descriptive Statistics.

Medicine	Mean	Median	Standard deviation	Variance	Mode
A	503.72	496.60	42.86	1837.07	414.02
B	214.23	213.81	51.64	2667.63	94.05

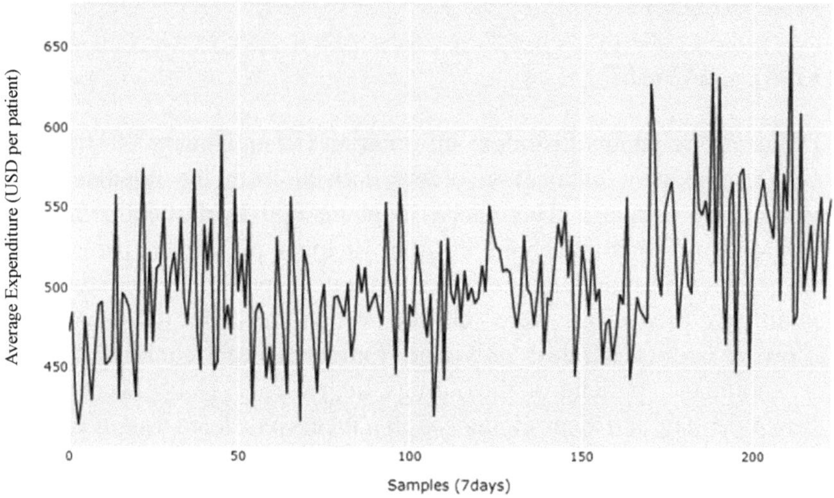

FIGURE 11.4 The behavior of expenditure made by patients for medication A.

The boxplot in Figure 11.6 shows the descriptive analysis of medications A and B expenditure. In medication A, some outliers are observed in the 75th percentile, corresponding to the daily average of instances far from the rest of the values. In the medication B boxplot, the median is located at the center of the box, representing the symmetric distribution. In medication A, 50% of the instances of the expense values are between 477 and 531. The dimensions of the box are determined by the distance of the interquartile range with a value of 54. Similarly, 50% of the spending values in the box of medication B are centered between 172 and 257 USD, with a median of 213.81 and an interquartile range of 85.

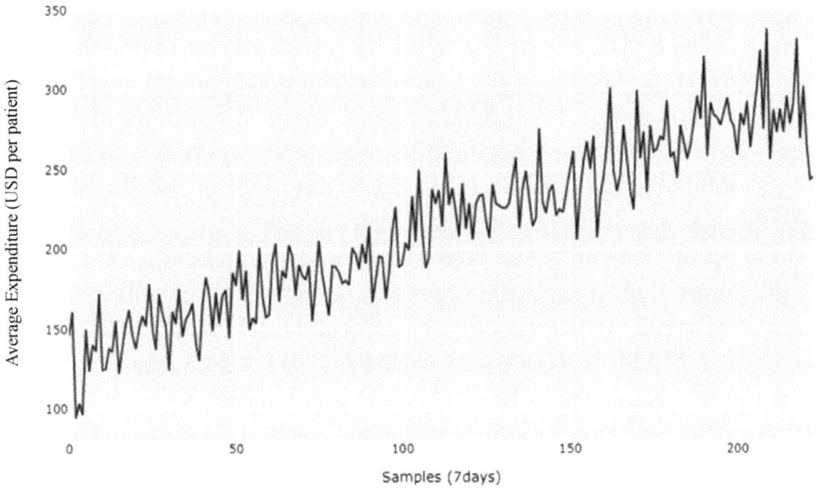

FIGURE 11.5 The behavior of expenditure made by patients for medication B.

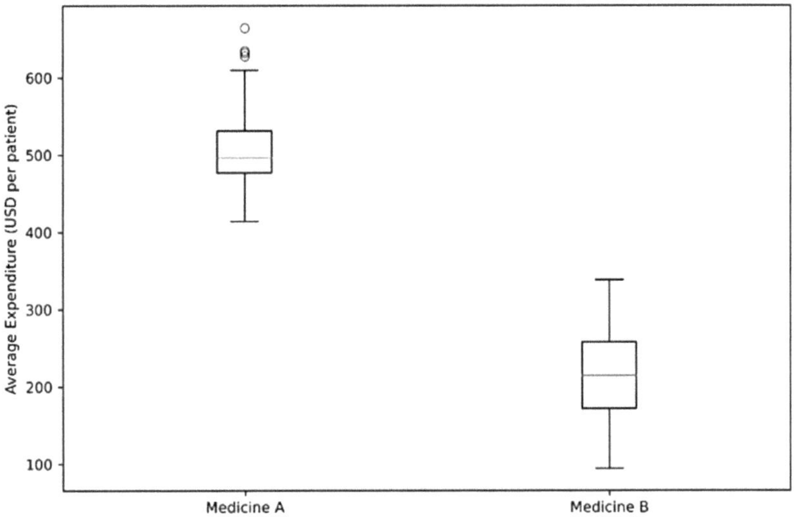

FIGURE 11.6 Described analysis of medication A and B expenditure.

11.4.3 EXPERIMENTAL RESULTS

Table 11.3 shows the values obtained in the RMSE, MAE, MAPE, and RMSLE metrics by the four DL models in the training phase for both medicines. The encoder–decoder LSTM model obtained the best performance in the RMSE metric for medicine A with a value of 46.00 using the data selected for the training stage of the inference model. In addition, it is observed that the CNN-LSTM model obtains values in the five metrics very close to the results obtained by the encoder–decoder LSTM model in its training stage (48.43, 36.53, 7.36, and 0.09 in the RMSE, MAE, MAPE, and RMSLE measurements, respectively).

On the other hand, the stacked LSTM model achieves the best measurement values of drug expenditure prediction in the training phase, using the dataset of medicine B (see Table 11.3), with an RMSE of 24.04, an MAE of 19.26, a MAPE of 10.09, and an RMSLE of 0.12. One aspect observed in the results displayed in Table 11.3 is that the CNN-LSTM model obtains a value of 24.08 in the RMSE metric; likewise, the encoder-decoder LSTM model obtains an RMSE of 24.59. Hence, both models have a very close learning capacity to the stacked LSTM model. In the case of the MAE and MAPE metrics, the encoder-decoder LSTM model obtains close values to those reached by the stacked LSTM model, but with a minimal difference, it is followed by the CNN-LSTM model.

TABLE 11.3 Results of DL Models during Training Stage.

Model	Medicine	RMSE	MAE	MAPE	RMSLE
LSTM	A	88.77	78.75	15.56	0.15
	B	34.29	28.64	14.37	0.20
Stacked LSTM	A	51.23	38.82	7.68	0.10
	B	24.04	19.26	10.09	0.12
CNN-LSTM	A	48.43	36.53	7.36	0.10
	B	24.08	19.56	10.21	0.13
Encoder–decoder LSTM	A	46.00	35.65	7.31	0.09
	B	24.59	19.53	10.10	0.12

Table 11.4 shows the results obtained in the testing stage of the four DL models. The encoder–decoder LSTM model acquired the lowest value in the RMSE error metric of 66.72 when predicting the expenditure of drug A. The model based on this network architecture achieves reliable performance compared to the result achieved by the model based on the LSTM neural network. Figure 11.7 shows the prediction overtime of the encoder–decoder LSTM model. It is observed that the behavior of the

prediction line follows the same behavior as the original data line. The blue line indicates the real value, and the red indicates the predicting value.

TABLE 11.4 Results of DL Models during Testing Stage.

Model	Medicine	RMSE	MAE	MAPE	RMSLE
LSTM	A	108.66	94.69	17.00	0.18
	B	42.74	37.16	12.87	0.17
Stacked LSTM	A	74.98	60.81	11.08	0.13
	B	31.26	25.39	8.78	0.11
CNN-LSTM	A	72.94	55.90	10.43	0.14
	B	30.24	24.08	8.37	0.10
Encoder–decoder LSTM	A	66.72	50.58	9.50	0.12
	B	34.29	28.57	9.86	0.10

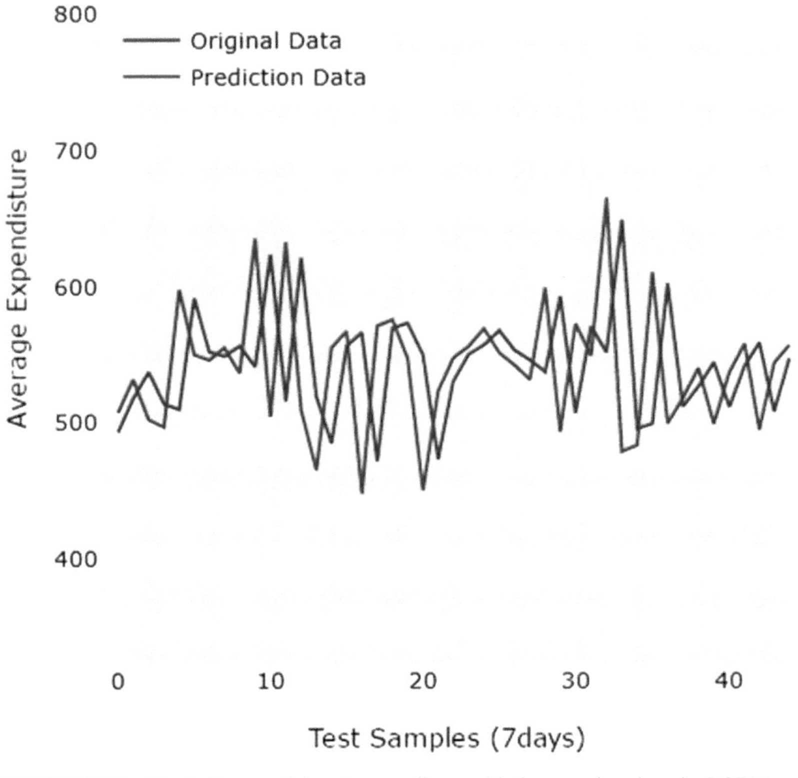

FIGURE 11.7 Prediction medicine A expenditure with the encoder–decoder LSTM model.

Figure 11.8 shows the expenditure prediction for the purchase of medication A, generated by the CNN-LSTM model. This model obtains values in metrics of 72.94, 55.90, 10.43, and 0.14 for RMSE, MAE, MAPE, and RMSLE, respectively, which are very close to the metrics achieved by the encoder–decoder LSTM model (see Table 11.4). Figure 11.8 shows similar behavior in patients' spending prediction to that observed in Figure 11.7. The main differences between the expenditure predictions of medication A generated by the two models can be seen when comparing Figures 11.7 and 11.8 in weeks 7–9, 21–26, and 36–40.

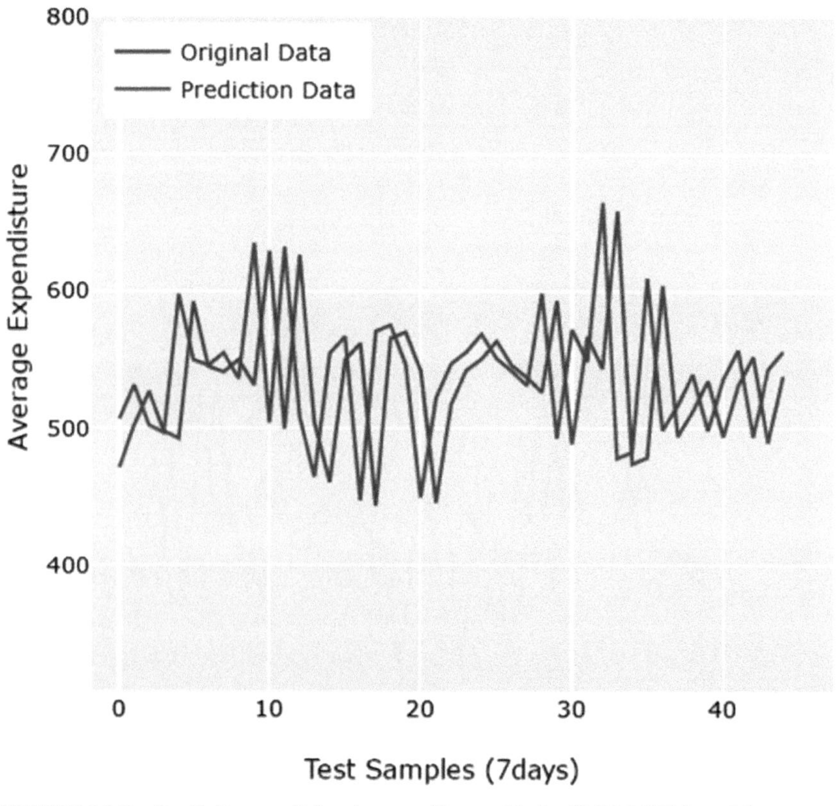

FIGURE 11.8 Prediction medicine A expenditure with the CNN-LSTM model.

In the results of the prediction of the expenditure of medication B, the best metrics were obtained by the CNN-LSTM model with an RMSE equal to 30.24, a MAE of 24.08, a MAPE of 8.37, and an RMSLE of 0.10

(see Table 11.4). The stacked LSTM model obtained values in its metrics very close to the CNN-LSTM model, with an RMSE of 31.26, a MAE of 25.39, a MAPE of 8.78, and an RMSLE of 0.11. This behavior can be seen in Figures 11.9 and 11.10, which show the prediction of drug B expenditure over time generated by the CNN-LSTM and stacked LSTM models, respectively. The prediction obtained from the test data follows the behavior identified for the original data of medicine B. The differences between the model predictions can be observed in weeks 5–10, 23–26, and 32–37. This difference can be observed in the separation between the real data line and the predicted data line in those weeks (see Figure 11.10).

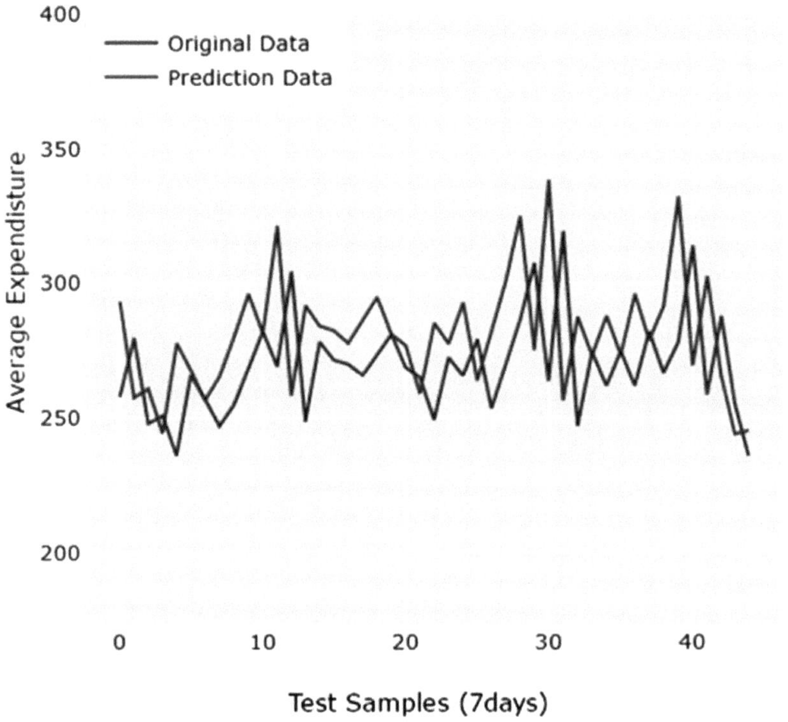

FIGURE 11.9 Prediction medicine B expenditure with the CNN-LSTM model.

11.5 CONCLUSIONS

The main objective of this research was to evaluate the performance of LSTM, stacked LSTM, CNN-LSTM, and encoder–decoder LSTM-based

DL architectures. In addition, based on the results obtained, a comparison was made between these models to identify the model with the highest performance capacity to predict the costs of medicine to support the planning that patients diagnosed with the disease require permanent medication. To comply with the above, we proposed a methodology that guides the process to select the best inference model, enabling the preparation of the input data, the design and training of the neural network model, and the selection of the best prediction model for each architecture. The dataset is transformed into a time-series scheme, which facilitates the data interpretation and prediction by models based on DL.

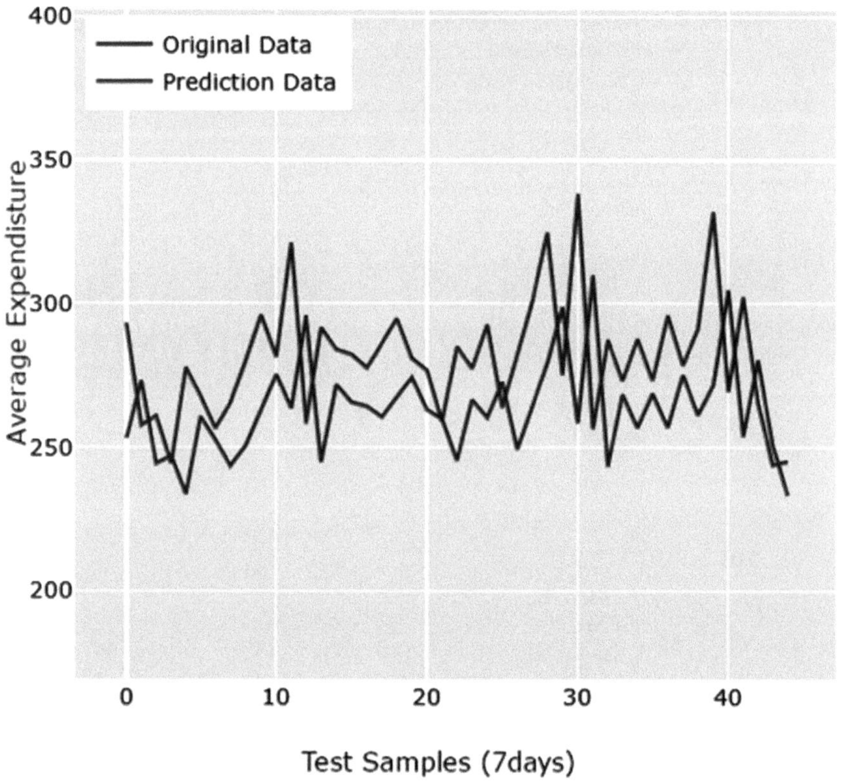

FIGURE 11.10 Prediction medicine B expenditure with the stacked LSTM model.

On the one hand, the best performance in the error metrics for medication A was identified from the encoder–decoder LSTM, followed by the CNN-LSTM and stacked LSTM models. On the other hand, the best performance for medicine B was observed in the CNN-LSTM model, followed by the performance obtained by the stacked LSTM and the encoder–decoder LSTM models. Furthermore, medicine B's prediction results were much better than the performance values of medicine A. With the CNN-LSTM model, the lowest RMSE obtained was 30.24 on test data for medicine B. We obtained 66.72 RMSE for medicine A with the encoder–decoder LSTM model.

We use a dataset with historical patient refilled medication orders to evaluate our methods' predictive performance, considering the transactions carried out in 1565 days. The proposed approach allowed us to know the feasibility of implementing methods based on DL to predict medical expenditure. The results achieved by these methods in our experimentation, considering the training and testing phases, allow us to confirm with values in the acceptable metrics for use in the problem posed in the healthcare domain.

KEYWORDS

- **medicine expenditure**
- **prediction model**
- **deep learning**
- **LSTM**
- **CNN**

REFERENCES

1. Sittig, D. F.; Wright, A.; Coiera, E.; Magrabi, F.; Ratwani, R.; Bates, D. W.; Singh, H. Current Challenges in Health Information Technology Related Patient Safety. *Health Inform. J.* **2020,** *26* (1), 181–189. DOI: 10.1177/1460458218814893.
2. Chen, S.-H.; Wen, P.-C.; Yang, C.-K. Business Concepts of Systemic Service Innovations in e-Healthcare. *Technovation* **2014,** *34* (9), 513–524. DOI: 10.1016/j.technovation.2014.03.002.
3. Negash, S.; Musa, P.; Vogel, D.; Sahay, S. Healthcare Information Technology for Development: Improvements in People's Lives through Innovations in the Uses of

Technologies. *Inf. Technol. Dev.* **2018,** *24* (2), 189–197. DOI: 10.1080/02681102.2018.1422477.

4. Soleimani-Roozbahani, F.; Rajabzadeh Ghatari, A. R.; Radfar, R. Knowledge Discovery from a More than a Decade Studies on Healthcare Big Data Systems: A Scientometrics Study. *J. Big Data* **2019,** *6* (1), 1–15. DOI: 10.1186/s40537-018-0167-y.
5. Islam, M. S.; Hasan, M. M.; Wang, X.; Germack, H. D.; Noor-E-Alam, M. A Systematic Review on Healthcare Analytics: Application and Theoretical Perspective of Data Mining. *Healthcare (Basel)* **2018,** *6* (2). DOI: 10.3390/healthcare6020054.
6. Sousa, M. J.; Pesqueira, A. M.; Lemos, C.; Sousa, M.; Rocha, Á. Decision-Making Based on Big Data Analytics for People Management in Healthcare Organizations. *J. Med. Syst.* **2019,** *43* (9), 290. DOI: 10.1007/s10916-019-1419-x
7. Waring, J.; Lindvall, C.; Umeton, R. Automated Machine Learning: Review of the State-of-the-Art and Opportunities for Healthcare. *Artif. Intell. Med.* **2020,** *104*, 101822. DOI: 10.1016/j.artmed.2020.101822.
8. Lee, C.; Luo, Z.; Ngiam, K. Y.; Zhang, M.; Zheng, K.; Chen, G.; Ooi, B. C.; Yip, W. L. J. Big Healthcare Data Analytics: Challenges and Applications. In *Handbook of Large-Scale Distributed Computing in Smart Healthcare*; Springer: Cham, 2017; pp 11–41. DOI: 10.1007/978-3-319-58280-1_2.
9. Rose, S. Robust Machine Learning Variable Importance Analysis of Medical Conditions for Health Care Spending. *Health Serv. Res.* **2018,** *53* (5), 3836–3854. DOI: 10.1111/1475-6773.12848.
10. Shrestha, A.; Mahmood, A. Review of Deep Learning Algorithms and Architectures. *IEEE Access* **2019,** *7*, 53040–53065. DOI: 10.1109/ACCESS.2019.2912200.
11. Ismail Fawaz, H. I.; Forestier, G.; Weber, J.; Idoumghar, L.; Muller, P. A. Deep Learning for Time Series Classification: A Review. *Data Min. Knowl. Discov.* **2019,** *33* (4), 917–963. DOI: 10.1007/s10618-019-00619-1.
12. Pham, T.; Tran, T.; Phung, D.; Venkatesh, S. Predicting Healthcare Trajectories from Medical Records: A Deep Learning Approach. *J. Biomed. Inform.* **2017,** *69*, 218–229. DOI: 10.1016/j.jbi.2017.04.001.
13. Kaushik, S.; Choudhury, A.; Dasgupta, N.; Natarajan, S.; Pickett, L. A.; Dutt, V. Using LSTMs for Predicting Patient's Expenditure on Medications. In *Proceedings of the 2017 International Conference on Machine Learning and Data Science (MLDS)*; IEEE Computer Society: Noida, India, 2017; pp 120–127. DOI: 10.1109/MLDS.2017.9.
14. Baytas, I. M.; Xiao, C.; Zhang, X.; Wang, F.; Jain, A. K.; Zhou, J. Patient Subtyping Via Time-Aware LSTM Networks. In *Proceedings of the 23rd ACM SIGKDD International Conference on Knowledge Discovery and Data Mining. Acad. Med.*, Halifax; 2017; pp 65–74. DOI: 10.1145/3097983.3097997.
15. Li, Y.; He, Z.; Wang, H.; Li, B.; Li, F.; Gao, Y.; Ye, X. CraftNet: A Deep Learning Ensemble to Diagnose Cardiovascular Diseases. *Biomed. Signal Process. Control* **2020,** *62*, 102091. DOI: 10.1016/j.bspc.2020.102091.
16. Zhang, L.; Zhang, Y.; Wang, L.; Wang, J.; Liu, Y. Diagnosis of Gastric Lesions through a Deep Convolutional Neural Network. *Dig. Endosc.* **2021,** *33* (5), 788–796. DOI: 10.1111/den.13844.

17. Zeng, X.; Lin, S.; Liu, C.; Deep Learning, M.-V. Multi-View Deep Learning Framework for Predicting Patient Expenditure in Healthcare. *IEEE Open J. Comput. Soc.* **2021,** *2*, 62–71. DOI: 10.1109/OJCS.2021.3052518.
18. Kaushik, S.; Choudhury, A.; Natarajan, S.; Pickett, L. A.; Dutt, V. Medicine Expenditure Prediction via a Variance-Based Generative Adversarial Network. *IEEE Access* **2020,** *8*, 110947–110958. DOI: 10.1109/ACCESS.2020.3002346.
19. Kaushik, S.; Choudhury, A.; Sheron, P. K.; Dasgupta, N.; Natarajan, S.; Pickett, L. A.; Dutt, V. AI in Healthcare: Time-Series Forecasting Using Statistical, Neural, and Ensemble Architectures. *Front. Big Data* **2020,** *3*, 4. DOI: 10.3389/fdata.2020.00004.
20. Kaushik, S.; Choudhury, A.; Dasgupta, N.; Natarajan, S.; Pickett, L. A.; Dutt, V. Ensemble of Multi-Headed Machine Learning Architectures for Time-Series Forecasting of Healthcare Expenditures. In *Applications of Machine Learning*; Springer: Cham, 2020, pp 199–216. DOI: 10.1007/978-981-15-3357-0_14.

CHAPTER 12

COVID-19 Detection from Chest X-Ray Using a Customized Artificial Neural Network

VINAYAK TIWARI, AMIT SINGHAL, and NISCHAY DHANKHAR

Department of Electronics and Communication, Netaji Subhas University of Technology, New Delhi, Delhi, India

ABSTRACT

Coronavirus disease (COVID-19) has affected the whole world in the past one year with over 5 million deaths so far. Reverse transcription-polymerase chain reaction (RT-PCR) test is used for COVID-19 diagnosis, but it results in high number of false-negative cases. Since most of the hospitals have X-ray machines available, diagnosing disease through chest X-ray can reduce overdependence on RT-PCR tests, especially when cases are increasing at a faster rate. In this era of pandemics, automated procedure of classifying images with disease can save time and human effort. This chapter deals with such classification techniques and a comparison of performances of various machine learning classifiers. The proposed method includes separate head training by using a pretrained convolutional neural network called ResNet-50 to extract features from images. These features are passed to various classifiers, including, random forest, *k*-nearest neighbor, logistic regression, and artificial neural network (ANN). The proposed methodology using custom ANN achieves better results as compared to other classifiers, with classification accuracy of 95.5%, f1 score of 96% for COVID, and 95% for normal class.

Applied Intelligence for Medical Image Analysis. Aarti, Raju Pal, Mukesh Saraswat, & Himanshu Mittal (Eds.)

12.1 INTRODUCTION

Coronavirus disease (COVID-19) disease is caused by SARS-COV-2 virus. COVID-19, a global pandemic, has taken lives of more than 5 million people across the globe. The whole world has suffered but the majorly impacted nations are USA, UK, India, Italy, Brazil, Russia, France, Iran, and Australia, where COVID-19 second wave has also been witnessed in the past one year. It is a viral disease and hence is contagious. Singhal et al.[1] had predicted the possible surge in COVID-19 cases in future that can help health-care sector to do necessary preparations in terms of proper treatment of patients. Effect of particulate matter on the spread of cases is analyzed by Singhal et al.[2] and the differences among the rate of spread across various regions are studied by Agarwal et al.[3]

However, it is also equally important to curb COVID-19 spread by early detection. Early detection of this disease by examining chest X-ray of the patient can become a lifesaving step. The reverse transcription-polymerase chain reaction (RT-PCR) test, used for diagnosis, not only has high false-negative rates, but it also depends upon how the sample is collected. This whole process requires human intervention and is time-consuming as well. Failure in reliable early detection of COVID-19 disease risks the chances of spreading the disease to healthy patients and may also lead to death of the patient.

X-ray scans are a useful source of reliable detection using radiographic features in the lungs of patients. Based on the radiographic changes, early diagnosis can be done accurately, even in patients who have been detected COVID negative after RT-PCR test. For COVID-19 prediction, Mishra et al.[4] have done their research using Dense-Net-based convolutional neural network (CNN). Jaiswal et al.[5] used a similar approach claiming that DenseNet201 is giving the best results. Shrinjal et al.[6] did their experiments on DarkCovidNet using X-ray images that gave 87% accuracy. Abdulmunim et al.[7] had also used X-ray images and got an accuracy of 85.58%. The proposed method of classification in this study gave better results on X-ray images compared to the abovementioned works.

This chapter is arranged as follows: Section 12.2 gives the details of the dataset used. Section 12.3 discusses the proposed method, CNN architecture, ResNet-50, and separate head learning approach. Section 12.4 provides the results of experiments and Section 12.5 concludes the chapter.

12.2 DATASET

BIMCV COVID-19+ dataset[8] is a publicly available dataset prepared by Valencian Regional Medical Image Bank (BIMCV). It contains chest X-ray and chest-computed tomography images of COVID-19-positive patients. For this chapter, a subset of BIMCV COVID-19+ dataset has been used that is available on the following link: https://www.kaggle.com/tawsifurrahman/covid19-radiography-database. This dataset has 3616 COVID-19-positive chest X-ray images, 10,192 normal chest X-ray images, 6012 lung opacity (non-COVID lung infection), and 1345 viral pneumonia X-ray images. Figure 12.1 shows sample X-ray images from the above-mentioned dataset.

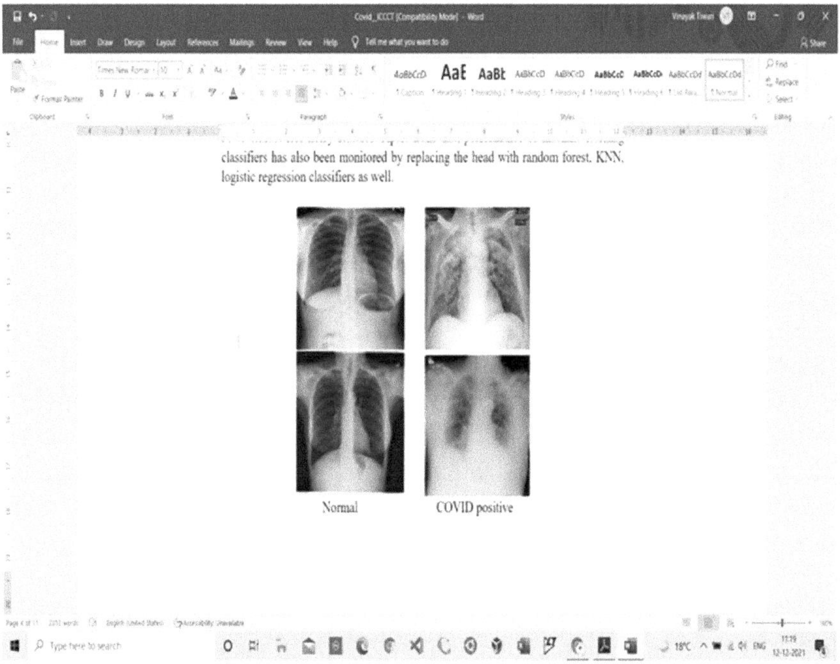

FIGURE 12.1 Chest X-rays of COVID-negative and -positive patients.

12.3 PROPOSED METHOD

In this chapter, a pretrained CNN model has been used to extract features from images. The pretrained CNN used in this study is ResNet-50[9] that has been trained on ImageNet dataset.[10] The X-ray images have been passed through this CNN and features have been extracted from the very last layer of CNN. The actual ANN layers of pretrained ResNet-50 also known as the top layers have been clipped and have been replaced by other classifiers like customized ANN, *k*-nearest neighbor (KNN),[11] random forest, and logistic regression. This approach has been used here since the dataset is quite small to yield good results.

This chapter deals with a COVID-19 disease classification problem and hence gives out a proposed model to classify chest X-ray of COVID-19 positive and chest X-rays of a normal patient. Data have been split into testing and training sets and necessary image scaling is done. After this, a pretrained ResNet-50 model has been used and the images have been passed through it. The top layers or the head of ResNet consisting of ANN have been removed, since it is meant to classify 1000 classes and this chapter's aim is to do binary classification. Features from the last convolutional layer of ResNet-50 have been then taken out and then allowed to pass through classifier models. A customized ANN model as shown in Figure 12.2 has been placed at the head of ResNet-50 to classify images. Since 2D CNN models use images as inputs, they do not capture vital information present in the raw image features. To address this shortcoming, various 1D CNN and ANN architectures are experimented on the features extracted from the ResNet-50 model.

The proposed ANN architecture demonstrates effectiveness of utilizing temporal models. It leverages convolution blocks, several dense layers, batch normalization layers, and a dense head to capture varying patterns. First, the features extracted from the ResNet-50 model are passed in the convolution 1D block to capture hierarchical features. Those features are then flattened to make it compatible for using dense layers. These features are passed through a total of seven dense blocks whose nodes are ranging from 2048 to 64. Deep networks provide higher predictive power in most deep learning tasks; however, the depth of the model is limited due to vanishing/exploding gradient phenomena. Therefore, each dense block used comprises three layers: dense layer, batch normalization, and dropout. The addition of batch normalization and dropout led to better generalization of the model preventing it from overfitting. Lastly, a dense head with single node is used to generate sigmoid predictions.

12.3.1 CONVOLUTIONAL NEURAL NETWORKS AND RESNET-50

CNNs are the special types of neural networks that are best used in cases where images are involved. It is basically a network of convolution layers followed by ANN at the top of it for classification. Image is a 2D data; hence, the features at the end of CNN and at the input of ANN must be flattened out for classification using ANN. This is done by a flattening layer at the top of the network. Hence, it can be said that there are two blocks, the first block works as a feature extractor by using convolutional filtering operations. Every convolutional layer consists of image kernels that give out feature maps and transfer them to the next layer which are then normalized using activation function, commonly used is ReLu.[12] This function applies max(0, x) threshold. Max-pooling[13] or average pooling layers have been used for spatial dimension reduction of the received data. Finally, the last feature maps are then flattened out for a suitable input for the second block. The second block is ANN used for classification consisting of dense layers and a normalized exponential function sigmoid as shown in Equation 12.1 has been used for binary classification to normalize data in the range of 0–1. At the end, the output layer gives output of CNN with loss function and label.

$$f(x) = (1 + e^{-x}) - 1 \tag{12.1}$$

The ResNet model was the winner of the 2015 ImageNet challenge. It became popular as training extremely deep neural networks with 150+ layers became possible after its invention. Before its invention, it was not possible to train such deeper networks due to the problem of vanishing gradients. Vanishing gradient is a problem caused due to repeated multiplication of the gradient when it backpropagates and makes the gradient very small. This results in the network performance getting saturated or even degrades when the network goes deeper and deeper. In this study, ResNet-50 is used as a feature extractor as shown in Figure 12.3, with 50 network layers. Skip connections as shown in Figure 12.4 are the strength of ResNet-50 that tackles vanishing gradient problems by using shortcut paths to allow gradients to flow. It also ensures that the higher layer will perform equally good as the previous layer and not worse than them.

12.3.2 SEPARATE HEAD TRAINING

The entire ResNet-50 model trained from scratch requires good computational resources. Due to the small size of the dataset used for this chapter, training a neural network from scratch is not a good option as it compromises with the desired results. Therefore, to avoid these issues, a new technique has been used for better results. In separate head training, the feature embeddings generated from a CNN model are used as features for training a different artificial neural network (ANN) or machine learning model. In this technique, X-ray images and image-net pretrained weights are used in ResNet-50 to extract less noisy features. Apart from that, performance of machine learning classifiers has also been monitored by replacing the head with random forest, KNN, and logistic regression classifiers as well.

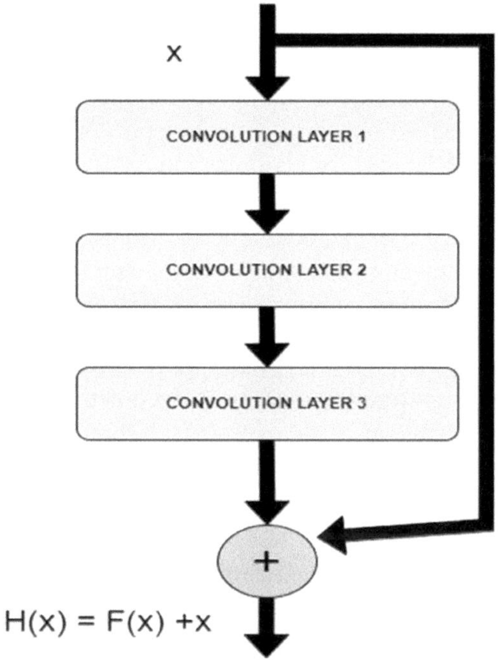

FIGURE 12.2 Skip connection.

12.4 RESULTS AND DISCUSSION

After classifying images using customized ANN model, for comparison purposes, KNN, random forest, logistic regression classifiers are also added one by one and their classification accuracy, area under curve (AUC) score, ROC curve, precision, recall, and f1-score values are discussed. Figure 12.5

shows the ROC curve while the confusion matrix of customized ANN is depicted in Figure 12.6.

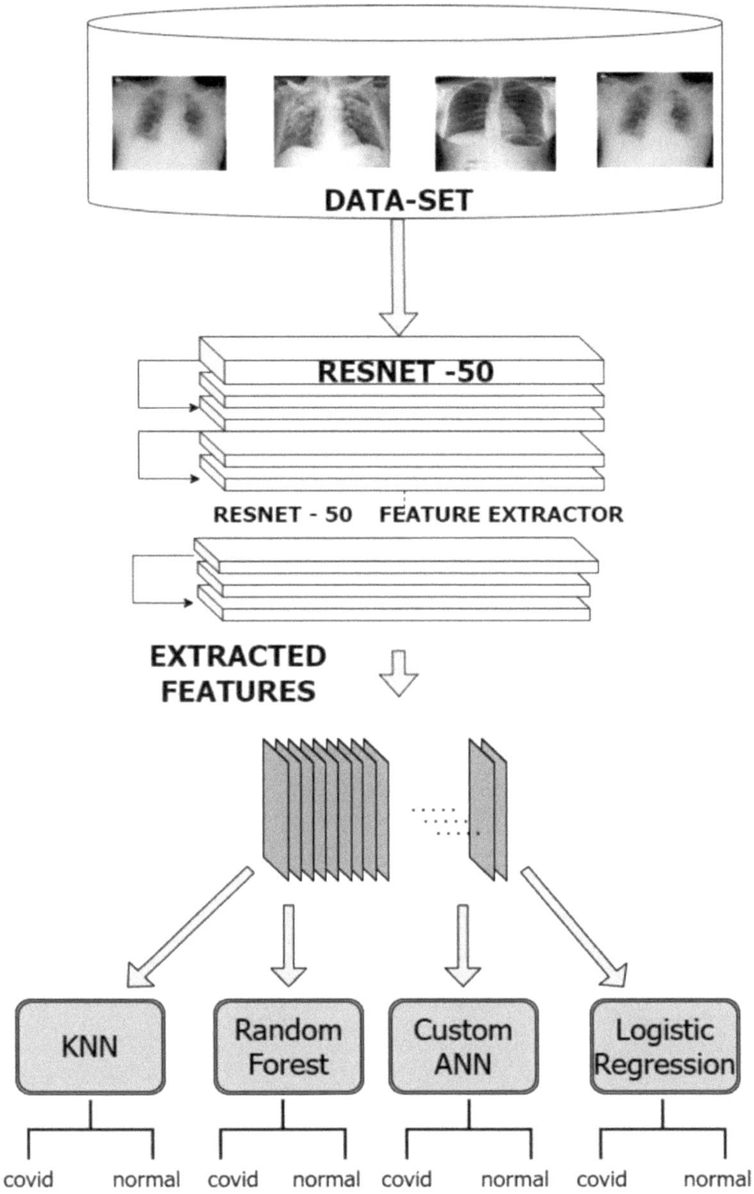

FIGURE 12.3 Proposed model architecture.

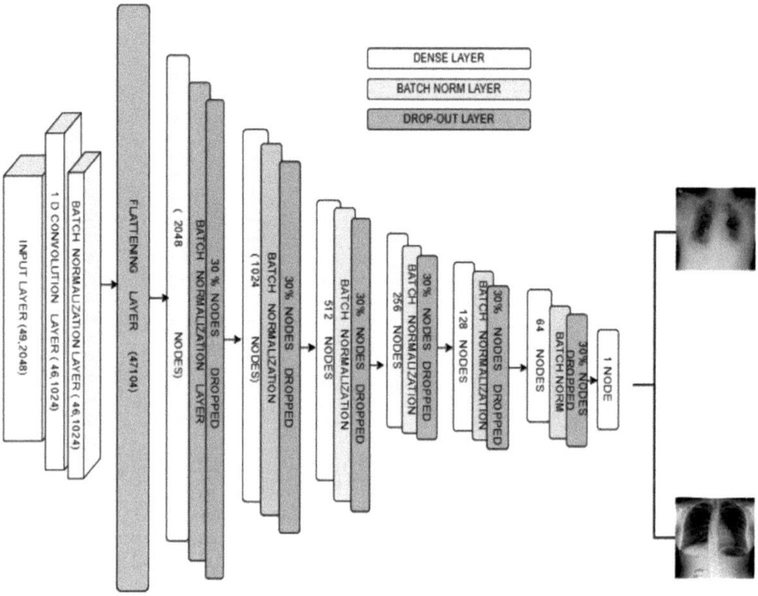

FIGURE 12.4 Customized ANN architecture.

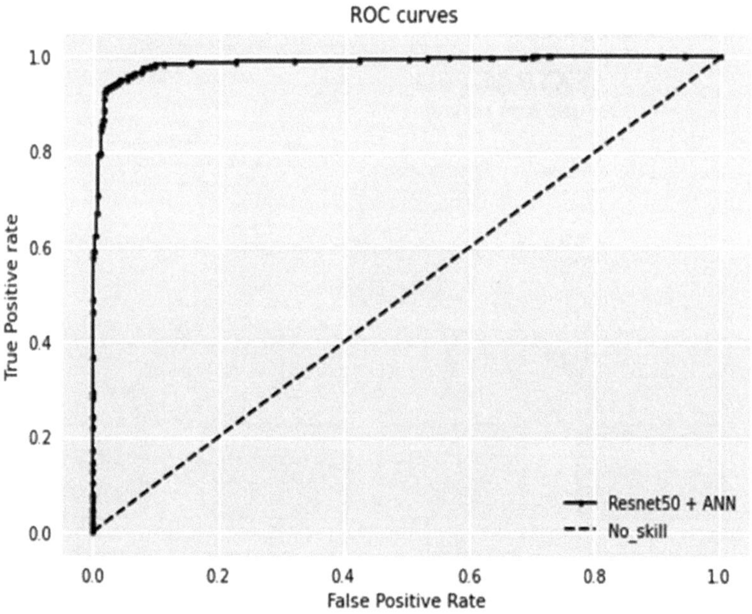

FIGURE 12.5 ROC curve of ResNet-50 with customized ANN.

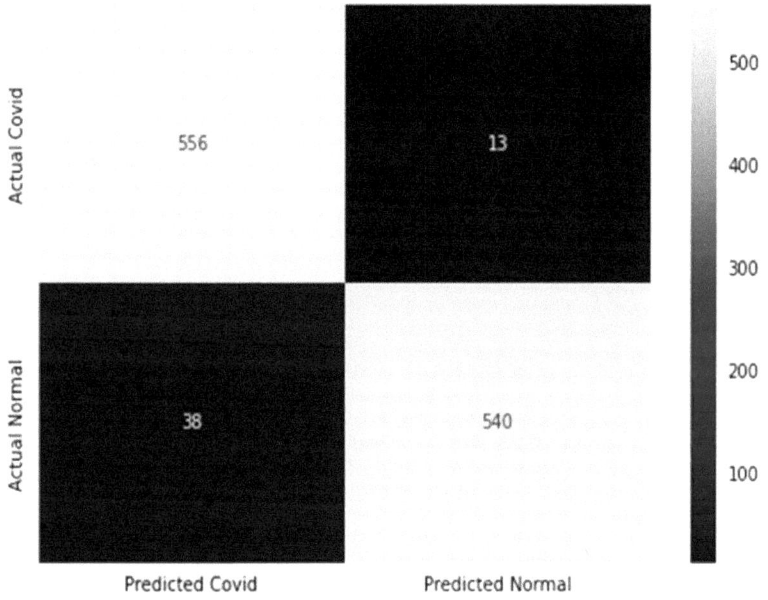

FIGURE 12.6 Confusion matrix of ResNet-50 with customized ANN.

For fitting customized ANN as a classifier, adam, stochastic gradient descent, and RMSprop optimizers with binary cross-entropy loss have been used. It has been found that adam optimizer converges fast as compared to other optimizers and is beneficial for adaptive learning. Threshold for binary classification is set to the optimal value of 0.13 since the model gives maximum AUC and accuracy at this point. Early stopping of model training is applied to prevent it from overfitting; hence, the model training stops after 12 epochs. The custom ANN model has shown AUC of 0.9877 and f1 score of 0.96 for COVID and 0.95 for normal class. Similarly, Figure 12.7 shows the ROC curves of other classifiers post-transfer learning. Table 1 gives the comparison of accuracy, f1 score, and AUC score of all classifiers.

12.5 CONCLUSION

This chapter highlights and establishes the utility of separate deeper ANN along with 1D CNNs to achieve high accuracy in detecting COVID using X-ray images. In comparison to 2D CNN models fine-tuned on the dataset, using a separate classifier head prevents the excessive need of computation without compromising the performance. The custom architecture of the proposed ANN is highly robust on the unseen data. Through this chapter, deep learning's potential in X-ray images with the usage of 1D CNN and ANN has been shown and gives out the best results compared to other machine learning classifiers with classification accuracy of 95.5%, f1 score of 96% for COVID and 95% for normal class, and AUC of 98.77%, hence eliminating the problem of false negatives in COVID-19 disease detection.

TABLE 12.1 Comparison of Different Classifiers.

Classifier	f1 score (%) COVID	f1 score (%) Normal	Accuracy (%)	AUC score (%)
Custom ANN	96	95	95.50	98.77
Logistic regression	94	93	94	98.70
KNN	87	84	86.01	85.60
Random forest	90	90	90	95.8

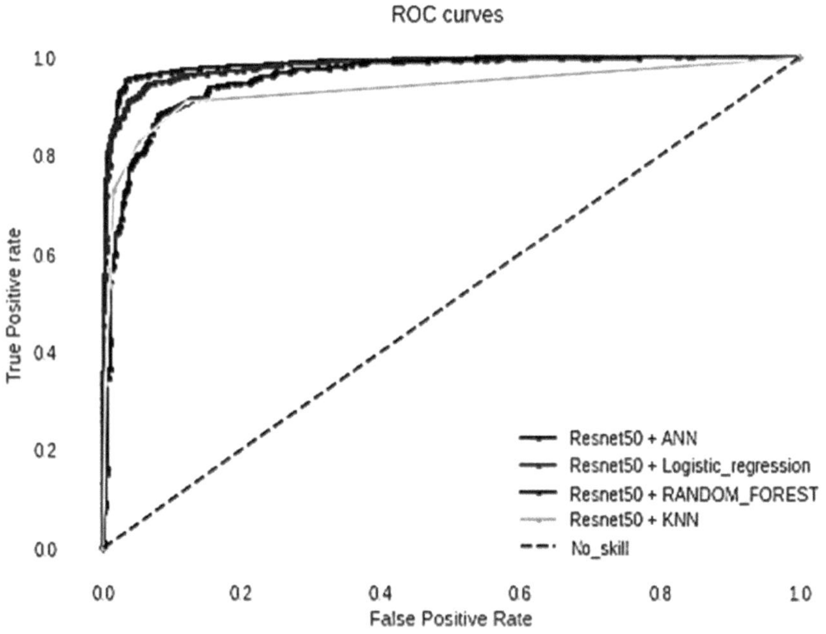

FIGURE 12.7 Comparison of ROC curves of various classifiers.

KEYWORDS

- **artificial neural network (ANN)**
- **convolution neural network (CNN)**
- ***k*-nearest neighbor (KNN)**
- **ResNet-50**

REFERENCES

1. Singhal, A.; Singh, P.; Lall, B.; Joshi, S. D. Modeling and Prediction of COVID-19 Pandemic Using Gaussian Mixture Model. *Chaos Solitons Fract.* **2020,** *138*, 110023. DOI: 10.1016/j.chaos.2020.110023.
2. Singhal, A.; et al. Ambient Fine Particulate Matter and COVID-19 in India. In *International Conference on Machine Intelligence and Signal Processing*, 2021.
3. Agarwal, M.; Singhal, A.; Patial, M.; Lall, B. Prediction of COVID-19 Cases and Attribution to Various Factors across Different Geographical Regions. In *International Conference on Innovations in Computational Intelligence and Computer Vision*, 2021.
4. Mishra, A. K.; Das, S. K.; Roy, P.; Bandyopadhyay, S. Identifying COVID-19 from Chest CT Images: A Deep Convolutional Neural Networks Based Approach. *J. Healthc. Eng.* **2020,** *2020*, 8843664. DOI: 10.1155/2020/8843664.
5. Jaiswal, A.; Gianchandani, N.; Singh, K. V.; Kaur, M. Classification of the COVID-19 Infected Patients Using densenet201 Based Deep Transfer Learning. *J. Biomol. Struct. Dyn.* **2020,** *39* (15), 5682–5689.
6. Shrinjal, S.; Piyush, S.; Aman, G.; Dinesh Kumar, V. CNN Based COVID-Aid: COVID 19 Detection Using Chest X-ray. In *International Conference on Computing Methodologies and Communication*, 2021.
7. Abdulmunim, A.; Nimat Saleem, N. Intelligent Tool for Detecting COVID-19 Using Convolutional Neural Network Based on Both CT and X-Ray Lung Images. *AIP Conf. Proc.* **2021,** *2404* (1). DOI: 10.1063/5.0068889.
8. de la Iglesia Vayá, M.; Saborit-Torres, J. M.; Serrano, J. A. M.; Oliver-Garcia, E.; Pertusa, A.; Bustos, A.; Cazorla, M.; Galant, J.; Barber, X.; Orozco-Beltrán, D.; García-García, F.; Caparrós, M.; González, G.; Salinas, J. M. BIMCV COVID-19+: A Large Annotated Dataset of RX and CT Images from COVID-19 Patients. *IEEE Dataport*. **2020**. DOI: 10.21227/w3aw-rv39.
9. He, K.; Zhang, X.; Ren, S.; Sun, J. Deep Residual Learning for image Recognition. In *Proceedings of the IEEE Conference on Computer Vision and Pattern Recognition*, 2016; pp 770–778.
10. Deng, J.; Dong, W.; Socher, R.; Li, L.; Li, K.; Fei-Fei, L. ImageNet: A Large-Scale Hierarchical Image Database. In *IEEE Conference on Computer Vision and Pattern Recognition*, 2009; pp 248–255. DOI: 10.1109/CVPR.2009.5206848(2009).

11. Guo, G.; Wang, H.; Bell, D.; Bi, Y.; Greer, K. An *k*NN Model-Based Approach and Its Application in Text Categorization. In *Computational Linguistics and Intelligent Text Processing*; Gelbukh, A., Ed.; CICLing 2004 Lecture Notes in Computer Science; Springer: Cham, 2004; Vol 2945, pp 559–570. DOI: 10.1007/978-3-540-24630-5_69.
12. Agarap, A. F. Deep Learning Using Rectified Linear Units (RELU). *arXiv Preprint* **2018**. ArXiv:1803.08375.
13. Gholamalinezhad, H.; Khosravi, H. Pooling Methods in Deep Neural Networks: A Review. *arXiv* **2020**. arXiv:2009.07485.

CHAPTER 13

An Automated Deep Learning Approach to Classify ECG Signals Using AlexNet

NEELOFER SHAHEEN[1], MUDASSIR HASAN KHAN[2], and MOHAMMAD SARFRAZ[1,3]

[1]*Department of Electrical Engineering, Aligarh Muslim University, Aligarh, Uttar Pradesh, India*

[2]*Centre for Interdisciplinary Biomedical and Human Factors Engineering, Aligarh Muslim University, Aligarh, Uttar Pradesh, India*

[3]*Soft Computing Research Society, New Delhi, Delhi, India*

ABSTRACT

The automated categorization study of electrocardiogram signals (ECG) has become increasingly important in the clinical diagnosis of disease as the prevalence of cardiovascular problems has increased. A convolutional neural network (CNN)-based approach is suggested for categorizing ECG signals. The deep learning approach, which uses CNNs, can recognize ECG readings automatically without the need for trivial manual feature extractions, but they require a lot of attention. In this study, we have used deep learning to classify and detect cardiac arrhythmia via AlexNet, one of the prominent pretrained CNNs. The proposed CNN model for cardiac arrhythmia classification consists of 25 layers, and spectrograms were used as input images to the CNN model. The experimental results show that the proposed technique achieves a promising classification accuracy, specificity, sensitivity, precision, and F1 score of more than 99%, outperforming several common ECG classification methods. The

Applied Intelligence for Medical Image Analysis. Aarti, Raju Pal, Mukesh Saraswat, & Himanshu Mittal (Eds.)

hyperparameters, that is, the epoch size and the minimum batch size, were varied, but despite several variations, the results were remarkable.

13.1 INTRODUCTION

An electrocardiogram (ECG) is a noninvasive procedure that records the electrical activities of the heart and can be used to detect a range of issues. Arrhythmic heartbeat classification within an ECG signal is often a difficult and time-consuming task for a clinician; as a result, hand-annotating such heartbeats is prone to inaccuracy. This requires the use of real-time automatic heartbeat classification algorithms capable of reliably diagnosing arrhythmic heartbeats. Deep learning–based algorithms, such as deep convolutional neural networks (CNNs), have recently been presented as a way to automatically extract information and increase ECG beat categorization accuracy. Image classification and segmentation,[6,16] landmark detection,[21] object identification,[2] face detection and recognition,[9,28] voice recognition,[11,15] and tongue processing are just a few of the disciplines where deep learning techniques have lately shown promise. The most significant advantage of deep learning methods is that they do not require a separate feature extraction step by human experts; instead, deep learning models perform feature extraction automatically and implicitly thanks to their powerful data learning capabilities and flexible processing architectures.

Deep learning features, according to some research, are more informative than expert features for ECG data. Deep learning algorithms outperform traditional methods in a range of ECG analysis applications, including disease identification and sleep staging. ECG data can teach cardiologists a lot about the heart's rhythm and function. As a result, its evaluation can be used to diagnose and treat a wide range of heart problems.[1]

While CNNs are useful when dealing with large amounts of data, they are prone to overfitting when dealing with datasets with little amounts of data. Using CNNs' pretrained networks on very big datasets and transferring the data to another categorization assignment with less training data is a common method recently adopted in the machine learning field. We propose that these models can be used to develop a reliable feature representation from recorded ECG training set in this work. Because the pretrained CNN employs RGB visuals and the ECG signals are raw vectors, we propose converting the ECG signals to spectrograms using the short-time Fourier transform (STFT). STFT was chosen because of its capacity to analyze ECG signals. The image-like input is then fed into the pretrained CNN, which generates the matching CNN features. The results suggest that the recommended technique improves accuracy more effectively.[17,19,22,23,32]

13.2 LITERATURE SURVEY

In 2021, some researchers[5] developed an approach that uses ECG signals to classify fall and no-fall events using pretrained CNNs' AlexNet and GoogLeNet. Eight volunteers were used in the study to get ECGs for both falling and nonfalling situations. The signals are preprocessed with an elliptical filter to remove signal noises like baseline drift and power-line interface. By applying a continuous wavelet transform (CWT) to filtered ECG data, feature extractors such as frequency-time representations were generated. The neural network used these images as inputs, and the first model achieved a substantial validation accuracy of 98.08%. The trained model can distinguish ECGs with a fall activity from ECGs without a fall activity with a 98.02% accuracy. In order to evaluate the robustness of the proposed approach, this experimental dataset was augmented with two different publicly accessible datasets. The second model can categorize fall, everyday activities, and no activities with a 98.44% accuracy.

In 2021,[30] work was done where patients with occasional heart arrhythmia benefit from remote checking gadgets that can be worn or embedded since they can consistently screen heart movement. To classify crude ECG accounts, they utilize profound convolutional neural networks (CNN). In any case, preparing CNNs for ECG grouping as often as possible necessitates a critical number of commented-on information, which can be expensive. They involved move figuring out how to resolve this issue in this review. To start, they preprepared CNNs utilizing the biggest freely accessible informational collection of ceaseless crude ECG signals. Utilizing a little informational index, the organizations are adjusted for the characterization of atrial fibrillation (AF), the most continuous heart arrhythmia. They show that pretraining further develops CNN execution on the goal task by up to 6.57%, successfully bringing down the quantity of comments expected to accomplish a similar degree of execution as undeveloped CNNs. They explore both directed and unaided pretraining approaches.

In a work done in 2020,[25] authors put their focus on detecting cardiac arrhythmia in the shortest possible period to prevent abrupt and premature deaths. The ECG signal is studied in this study using a comprehensive methodology. The lowest, maximum, mean, standard deviation, and median were the primary features retrieved in the proposed study. In the study, researchers examined 45 ECG records from the MIT BIH arrhythmia database and the MIT BIH noise stress test database. The suggested model is 96.7% accurate overall, 96.7% sensitivity, and 100% positive predictive value.

A research work carried out in 2020[14] developed an image classification approach based on upgraded AlexNet which is suggested to address the problems that the classic CNN has many parameters and a large proportion of completely connected parameters. This technique enhances classic AlexNet by including a deep convolution layer, categorizing the photos according to their whole connection layer. To test the categorization, the Cifar-10 data set was used. The findings show that the strategy not only decreases the number of parameters but also improves their quality, not only increasing the proportion of the whole connection layer, but it was also improving categorization as compared to AlexNet.

Similarly, work done in 2019[18] proposed research to provide a deep learning–based solution that can replace manual features of existing automatic AF classification methods which are based on hand-crafted features. AF is a type of heart arrhythmia that affects people all over the world. The majority of CNN-dubbed AlexNet was built using 5655 single-lead ECG records. They first created a spectrogram for all 30 signals and then used the CWT to convert them to RGB images, which were then fed into AlexNet and trained with a variety of settings. The results of the study reveal that the strategy beats all other methods, with a state-of-the-art accuracy of 97.9% and an F1 score of 98.82%, as well as higher overall sensitivity (98.9%) and specificity (90.7%).

In another article,[10] the authors proposed an effective ECG arrhythmia classification approach based on a deep two-dimensional CNN, which has lately demonstrated remarkable pattern recognition ability. As input data for the CNN classifier, each ECG beat was converted into a two-dimensional gray-scale image. In addition, they compared their suggested classifier against AlexNet and VGGNet, two well-known CNN models.

The classifier was evaluated using ECG records from the MIT-BIH arrhythmia database. As a result, their classifier had an average accuracy of 99.05% and a sensitivity of 97.85%. At the assessment, 10-fold cross-validation was used to precisely validate our CNN classifier, with each ECG recording being used as test data. The proposed CNN classifier, when used with modified ECG pictures, achieves outstanding classification accuracy without any manual ECG signal preprocessing such as noise filtering, feature extraction, or feature reduction, according to their results.

In 2018, Yildirim et al.[31] planned another strategy in light of deep learning of how to effectively and immediately group cardiovascular arrhythmias. For one lead, the people behind exploration gathered 1000 ECG signal pieces from 45 people from the MIT-BIH arrhythmia information base. (All things considered, multiple times less orders/investigations.) An exhaustive start-to-finish structure was built rather than the hand-created include extraction and choice utilized in old strategies. The plan of a novel 1D-CNN model was their key commitment (1D-CNN). The proposed strategy is (1) effective, (2) fast (real-time categorization), (3) simple, and (4) clear to execute (joined include extraction and determination, and characterization in one phase). For 17 heart arrhythmia problems (classes), deep 1D-CNN acquired a general acknowledgment exactness of 91.33% and an order time for every single example of 0.015 s.

Another work done by Pandey and Janghel[20] discussed that an 11-layer deep CNN model is used to classify the MIT-BIH arrhythmia database into five categories using the ANSI-AAMI criteria. He created a complete end-to-end structure of the classification approach in this CNN model and used it without the database's denoising process. The suggested new methodology has the primary benefit of reducing the number of categories and eliminating the need to detect and segment QRS complexes. Using the SMOTE methodology, the MIT-BIH database was intentionally used. To deal with the problem of minority classes and class imbalance, oversampling was used. The expanded ECG database was used to train the new CNN model, which was then evaluated on a real dataset. In comparison to the work stated in the literature, the developed CNN model outperforms the control model in terms of precision, recall, F-score, and total accuracy, according to the results. These findings also show that the 70:30 train–test data set achieves the highest performance accuracy of 98.30%.

Beforehand, a work[12] arranged 1.3 million high-goal photographs in the LSVRC-2010 ImageNet preparing set into 1000 separate classes. They prepared an immense, profound CNN. They accomplished top one and top five mistake paces of 39.7% and 18.9% on the test information, separately, which is fundamentally better compared to the earlier cutting-edge outcomes. Five convolutional layers, some of which are trailed by max-pooling layers, and two worldwide connected layers with a last 1000-way softmax, include the neural networks, which have 60 million boundaries and 500,000 neurons. They utilized nonsoaking neurons and an extremely effective GPU execution of convolutional nets to make preparing speed up. They utilized non-soaking neurons and an extremely effective GPU execution of convolutional nets to speed up preparation. They (Krizhevsky et al., 2012) utilized another regularisation methodology to lessen overfitting in the around-the-world associated layers, which was very successful.

13.3 DATASET DESCRIPTION

In this work, the MIT-BIH Arrhythmia Database[3,7] was used. Each of the 48 records in the MIT-BIH arrhythmia database is made up of 30 min ECG segments extracted from a 24-h recording of 47 different patients. From the total data, 21,010 s of ECG data was taken and categorized as normal and arrhythmia class. The arrhythmia class consisted of different types of arrhythmias such as left bundle branch block and right bundle branch block.

13.4 METHODOLOGY

In this work, initially, the MIT-BIH Arrhythmia Database as a whole was divided into two classes that are normal and arrhythmia. The data were converted into images known as spectrograms with the help of STFT. To begin with spectrograms, the data are digitally sampled in the time domain. The whole signal is then divided into several sections, and then Fourier transforms each section in order to calculate the magnitude of the frequency spectrum of each section. Furthermore, these frequency spectra are arranged so as to form spectrogram images.

The extraction and organization components of the convolutional neural system[26] are the most important. The spotlight extraction section is in charge of naturally removing relevant highlights from the ECG signals, while the other section is in charge of accurately defining signals utilizing the extricated highlights.

13.4.1 ECG PREPROCESSING

Baseline wandering, electromyography disturbance, and power line interference are just some of the noises that can occur; they often wreak havoc on clinically acquired ECG data, making it impossible to retrieve relevant information from an unprocessed signal. As a result, filtering is required before further signal processing. Because extra filtering can result in the loss of valuable information, we only eliminate the noise—baseline wandering, which has a major impact on ECG categorization.[8] Baseline drifting is caused by breathing or movement of the chest.[26] The baseline is removed using a bandpass filter in this case.

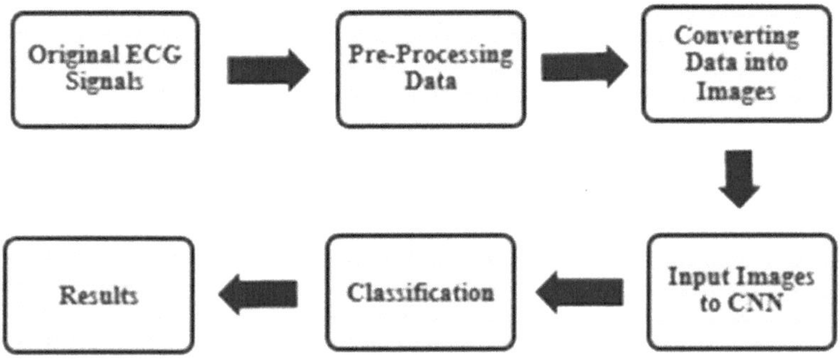

FIGURE 13.1 Flow diagram of ECG classification.

To preprocess the ECG signal, we use the following procedures:

- Set the normalization range of the ECG signal to zero to one.
- To ensure an even distribution, we have taken around 10,510 s of data for the normal class and 10,500 s of data for the arrhythmia class.
- Spectrogram images of a one-second window having 200 samples each were constructed, that is, we had 21,010 images for our study.
- Out of these spectrograms, 19,100 were used for training and validation, whereas 1910 were used for the testing.

13.4.2 ECG CLASSIFICATION BASED ON CNN

Artificial intelligence helps computer systems behave intelligently. Machine learning allows the software to learn on its own, but the learning features must be appropriately discovered and trained by the programmer. Deep learning, on the other hand, employs additional mathematics, neural networks, and processing to assist the computer in recognizing and generating correct and valuable results. CNN[22] is a deep learning concept that aims to extract signal/image data feature representations at multiple levels of computation. It comprises a progression of convolutional and pooling layers that substitute with completely associated layers. The convolutional layer is the fundamental structure square of CNN and addresses the design of profound models. The quantity of component maps delivered by this layer is administered by the quantity of channels utilized in the convolution layer. The learnable filters' feature maps are frequently sent to a nonlinear gating function like the rectified linear unit (ReLU).[27]

In addition, the activation function's output can be normalized to aid generalization. The feature map's data dimensions are reduced by the pooling layers, resulting in the only output from every block. Fully connected layers are utilized to execute high-level reasoning in the neural network after several convolutional and pooling layers, which is referred to as the classification phase at the output's conclusion. The last layer connects every neuron within the layer to all of the neurons from the previous layer. For categorization, we add a softmax layer to the end of this network.

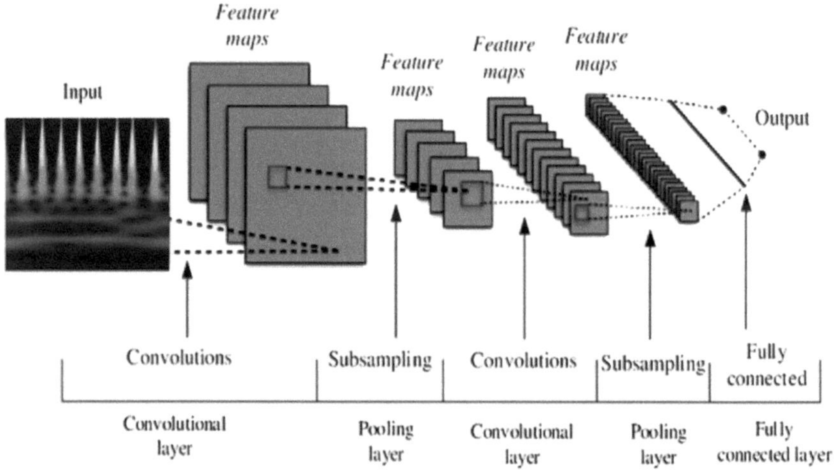

FIGURE 13.2 CNN architecture and convolutional neural network (CNN) taking ECG data input as image.

The learnable filters' feature maps are frequently sent to a nonlinear gating function like the ReLU.[24] The activation function, which can be linear or nonlinear, is a critical component of neural networks. One of the most important tools is the ReLU. In deep neural networks, it is the most fundamental and often used nonlinear activation function. It thrives in the vanishing gradient problem because its gradient value is either 0 or 1, and the mathematical formula is given as $f(x) = \max(0, x)$.

13.4.3 ALEXNET

FeiFei Li, a Stanford University professor, created ImageNet, a collection of annotated real-world objects. To study image recognition challenges, ImageNet organized an annual object classification competition called the ILSVRC. Though CNN's origins may be traced back to LeNet,[13] it was designed for certain purposes such as digit identification and was unable to provide a satisfactory result for all class pictures. When Alex Krizhevsky released a new image classification system with AlexNet, which won the ImageNet competition in 2012, this problem in CNN architecture was addressed.[4] AlexNet was designed by Alex Krizhevsky and is one of the contemporary CNN architectures. This pretrained network originally proposed in 2012 consists of a total of eight layers, in which the first five are convolution layers, and the remaining are fully connected layers. The latest AlexNet consisted of a total of 25 layers with a depth of 8 and 61 million parameters. It utilized the ReLUs instead of the standard tanh function and was able to cut down the computational time. Another technique it possesses is to take advantage of multiple GPUs available by dividing the total neurons among the GPUs to reduce the training time considerably. It also performs overlapped pooling to reduce the error. To overcome the overfitting problem, the model augmentation of the data was done, and certain neurons with predetermined probability were turned off in each iteration. The input image size for AlexNet must be 227*227*3.

13.5 RESULTS

13.5.1 TRAINING AND VALIDATION

In this work, deep learning pretrained network AlexNet used was trained with the help of spectrogram images; 19,100 spectrogram images were used for the training and validation purpose. The learning rate was adjusted to 0.0003, whereas the hyperparameters were tuned to get the best possible results. The epoch size was varied from 10 to 50 with a variation of 10 each time, whereas the minimum batch size was set to 16, 24, and 32 for each epoch size.

```
25x1 Layer array with layers:

 1   'data'    Image Input                   227x227x3 images with 'zerocenter' normalization
 2   'conv1'   Convolution                   96 11x11x3 convolutions with stride [4  4] and padding [0  0  0  0]
 3   'relu1'   ReLU                          ReLU
 4   'norm1'   Cross Channel Normalization   cross channel normalization with 5 channels per element
 5   'pool1'   Max Pooling                   3x3 max pooling with stride [2  2] and padding [0  0  0  0]
 6   'conv2'   Convolution                   256 5x5x48 convolutions with stride [1  1] and padding [2  2  2  2]
 7   'relu2'   ReLU                          ReLU
 8   'norm2'   Cross Channel Normalization   cross channel normalization with 5 channels per element
 9   'pool2'   Max Pooling                   3x3 max pooling with stride [2  2] and padding [0  0  0  0]
10   'conv3'   Convolution                   384 3x3x256 convolutions with stride [1  1] and padding [1  1  1  1]
11   'relu3'   ReLU                          ReLU
12   'conv4'   Convolution                   384 3x3x192 convolutions with stride [1  1] and padding [1  1  1  1]
13   'relu4'   ReLU                          ReLU
14   'conv5'   Convolution                   256 3x3x192 convolutions with stride [1  1] and padding [1  1  1  1]
15   'relu5'   ReLU                          ReLU
16   'pool5'   Max Pooling                   3x3 max pooling with stride [2  2] and padding [0  0  0  0]
17   'fc6'     Fully Connected               4096 fully connected layer
18   'relu6'   ReLU                          ReLU
19   'drop6'   Dropout                       50% dropout
20   'fc7'     Fully Connected               4096 fully connected layer
21   'relu7'   ReLU                          ReLU
22   'drop7'   Dropout                       50% dropout
23   ''        Fully Connected               3 fully connected layer
24   ''        Softmax                       softmax
25   ''        Classification Output         crossentropyex
```

FIGURE 13.3 AlexNet architecture.

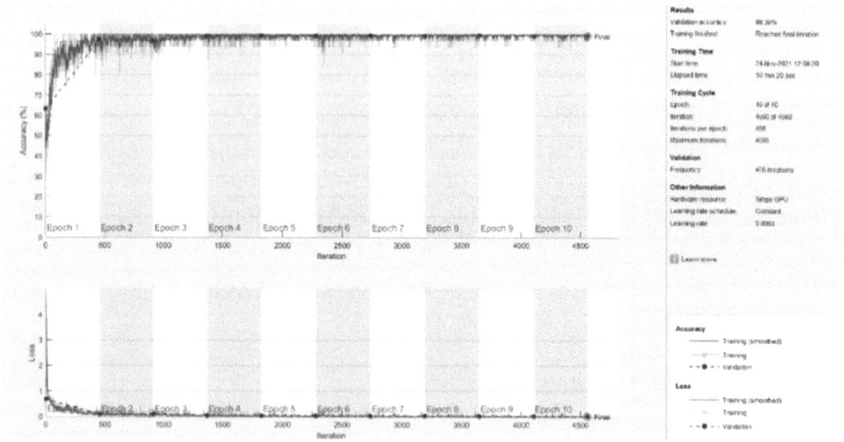

FIGURE 13.4 A sample of training and validation curve showing validation accuracy of 99.30% at epoch size of 10 and mini-batch size of 32.

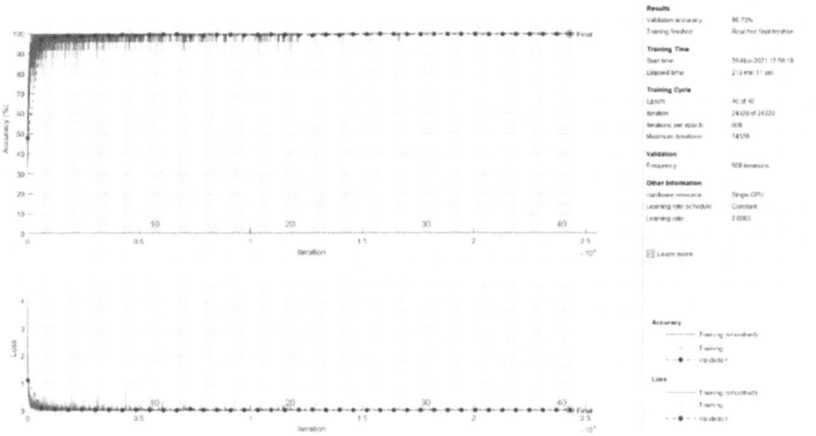

FIGURE 13.5 A sample of training and validation curve showing validation accuracy of 99.73% at epoch size of 40 and mini-batch size of 24.

13.5.2 TESTING

For testing, 10% of the training and validation data, that is, 1910 spectrogram images, were used. The testing was done, and the results were verified with the help of a confusion matrix. The evaluation was done in terms of true positive (TP), false positive (FP), true negative (TN), and false negative (FN). Furthermore, the results were indicated in terms of accuracy, precision, sensitivity, specificity, and F1 score.

$$\text{ACCURACY}\,(\%) = \frac{(\text{TP}+\text{TN})}{(\text{TN}+\text{TP}+\text{FN}+\text{FP})} \times 100 \tag{13.1}$$

$$\text{SENSITIVITY}\,(\%) = \frac{(\text{TP})}{(\text{TP}+\text{FN})} \times 100 \tag{13.2}$$

$$\text{SPECIFICITY}\,(\%) = \frac{(\text{TN})}{(\text{TN}+\text{FP})} \times 100 \tag{13.3}$$

$$\text{PRECISION}\,(\%) = \frac{(\text{TP})}{(\text{TP}+\text{FP})} \times 100 \tag{13.4}$$

$$\text{F1 SCORE} = \frac{(200\ \text{TP}^2)}{(101\ \text{TP}^2 + \text{TP}(\text{FP}+\text{FN}))} \tag{13.5}$$

$$\text{F1 SCORE} = 2 * \frac{(SENSITIVITY * PRECISION)}{(\text{SENSITIVITY} + \text{PRECISION})} \tag{13.6}$$

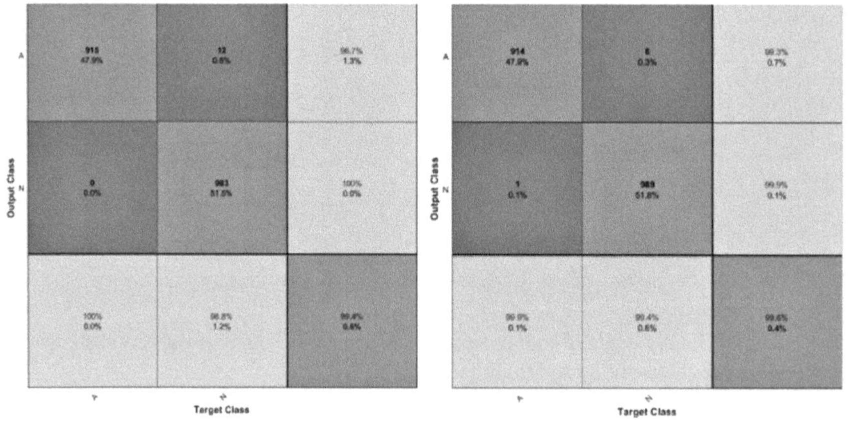

(a) (b)

FIGURE 13.6 Sample of confusion matrix (a) for epoch size of 30 and mini-batch size of 32 and (b) for epoch size of 40 and mini-batch size of 24, showing TP, TN, FP, and FN values which are further used to calculate testing accuracy, sensitivity, specificity, precision, and F1 score.

TABLE 13.1 Various Performance Parameters for Different Epoch Sizes at a Minimum Batch Size of 16.

Epoch size	Validation accuracy (%)	Testing accuracy (%)	Sensitivity (%)	Specificity (%)	Precision (%)	F1 score (%)
10	99.34	99.4	99.0	99.9	99.9	99.45
20	99.81	99.8	99.8	99.8	99.8	99.80
30	99.69	99.8	99.7	99.7	100	99.85
40	99.79	99.8	99.6	99.9	99.8	99.69
50	99.58	99.8	99.8	99.7	100	99.89

13.6 CONCLUSION

In this study, AlexNet was used to classify the ECG signals into normal and arrhythmia. The hyperparameters, that is, epoch size and mini-batch size, were varied in order to get the best combination which provides

TABLE 13.2 Various Performance Parameters for Different Epoch Sizes at a Minimum Batch Size of 24.

Epoch size	Validation accuracy (%)	Testing accuracy (%)	Sensitivity (%)	Specificity (%)	Precision (%)	F1 score (%)
10	99.15	99.5	99.3	99.8	99.8	99.55
20	99.38	99.9	99.9	100	100	99.95
30	99.65	99.8	99.6	100	100	99.79
40	99.73	99.6	99.4	99.9	99.9	99.65
50	99.43	99.7	99.7	99.8	99.7	99.70

TABLE 13.3 Various Performance Parameters for Different Epoch Sizes at a Minimum Batch Size of 32.

Epoch size	Validation accuracy (%)	Testing accuracy (%)	Sensitivity (%)	Specificity (%)	Precision (%)	F1 score (%)
10	99.30	99.4	98.8	100	100	99.39
20	99.26	99.7	99.7	99.8	99.8	99.75
30	99.73	99.9	99.8	100	100	99.89
40	99.61	99.7	99.6	99.9	99.7	99.65
50	99.38	99.5	99.3	99.7	99.9	99.59

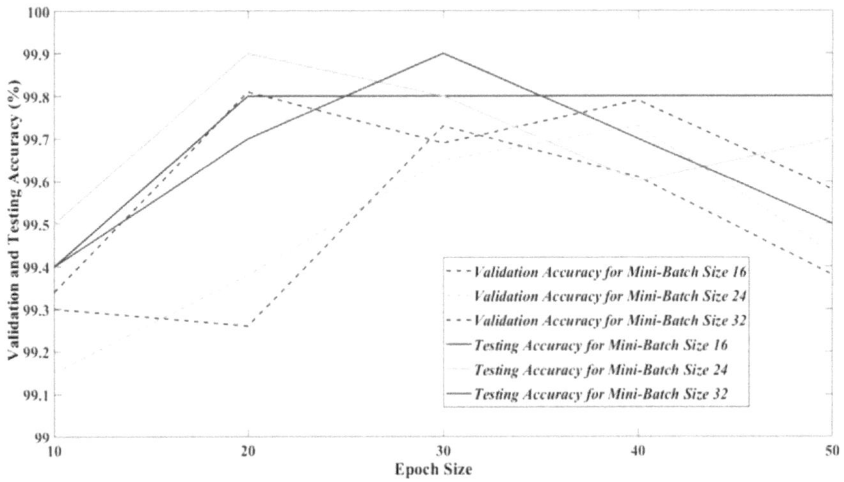

FIGURE 13.7 Graph showing the values of validation and testing accuracies (%) at the epoch size of 10, 20, 30, 40, and 50, respectively, for the three values of minimum batch size, that is, 16, 24, and 32.

promising results. As the training, validation, as well as testing was done, it was observed that the variation in the hyperparameters does not affect the accuracy to a greater extent. In each of the cases, we got validation as well as testing accuracy to be more than 99% with precision up to 100% in some cases. The thing which is getting affected by tuning these hyperparameters is the time taken for training and validation by the network. The epoch size of 10 and mini-batch size of 32 gives the validation accuracy of 99.3% taking 10 min and 20 s, while the combination of epoch size 40 and mini-batch size 24 provides 99.73% validation accuracy taking 213 min and 11 s. From here, we can conclude that this network, that is, AlexNet, gives promising results irrespective of the values of the hyperparameters.

KEYWORDS

- **cardiovascular disease**
- **convolution neural network**
- **ECG signal**
- **classification**
- **spectrogram**
- **AlexNet**

REFERENCES

1. Azizpour, H.; Razavian, A. S.; Sullivan, J.; Maki, A.; Carlsson, S. Factors of Transferability for a Generic Convnet Representation. *IEEE Trans. Pattern Anal. Mach. Intell.* **2016,** *38* (9), 1790–1802. DOI: 10.1109/TPAMI.2015.2500224.
2. Bai, J.; Wu, Y.; Zhang, J.; Chen, F. Subset Based Deep Learning for RGB-D Object Recognition. *Neurocomputing* **2015,** *165*, 280–292. DOI: 10.1016/j.neucom.2015.03.017.
3. Baim, D. S.; Colucci, W. S.; Monrad, E. S.; Smith, H. S.; Wright, R. F.; Lanoue, A.; Gauthier, D. F.; Ransil, B. J.; Grossman, W.; Braunwald, E. Survival of Patients with Severe Congestive Heart Failure Treated with Oral Milrinone. *J. Am. Coll. Cardiol.* **1986,** *7* (3), 661–670. DOI: 10.1016/s0735-1097(86)80478-8.
4. Bouaziz, B.; Chaari, L.; Batatia, H.; Quintero-Rincón, A. Epileptic Seizure Detection Using a Convolutional Neural Network. In *Digital Health Approach for Predictive,*

Preventive, Personalized and Participatory Medicine; Springer: Cham, 2019; pp 79–86. DOI: 10.1007/978-3-030-11800-6_9.

5. Butt, F. S.; La Blunda, L.; Wagner, M. F.; Schäfer, J.; Medina-Bulo, I.; Gómez-Ullate, D. Fall Detection from Electrocardiogram (ECG) Signals and Classification by Deep Transfer Learning. *Information* **2021,** *12* (2), 63. DOI: 10.3390/info12020063.
6. Gao, Z.; Wang, L.; Zhou, L.; Zhang, J. HEp-2 Cell Image Classification with Deep Convolutional Neural Networks. *IEEE J. Biomed. Health Inform.* **2017,** *21* (2), 416–428. DOI: 10.1109/JBHI.2016.2526603.
7. Goldberger, A. L.; L.; Amaral, L. A. N.; Glass, L.; Hausdorff, J. M.; Ivanov, P. Ch.; Mark, R. G.; Mietus, J. E.; Moody, G. B.; Peng, C.-K.; Stanley, H. E. PhysioBank, PhysioToolkit, and Physionet: Components of a New Research Resource for Complex Physiologic Signals. *Circulation* **2000,** *101* (23), e215–e220.
8. He, J.; Rong, J.; Sun, L.; Wang, H.; Zhang, Y.; Ma, J. A Framework for Cardiac Arrhythmia Detection from IoT-Based ECGs. *World Wide Web* **2020,** *23* (5), 2835–2850. DOI: 10.1007/s11280-019-00776-9.
9. Huang, Z.; Wang, R.; Shan, S.; Chen, X. Face Recognition on Large-Scale Video in the Wild with Hybrid Euclidean-and-Riemannian Metric Learning. *Pattern Recognit.* **2015,** *48* (10), 3113–3124. DOI: 10.1016/j.patcog.2015.03.011.
10. Jun, T. J.; Nguyen, H. M.; Kang, Daeyoun; Kim, D.; Kim, D.; Kim, Y.-H. ECG Arrhythmia Classification Using a 2-D Convolutional Neural Network. *ArXiv* **2018**. ArXiv:1804.06812.
11. Kiranyaz, S.; Ince, T.; Gabbouj, M. Real-Time Patient-Specific ECG Classification by 1-D Convolutional Neural Networks. *IEEE Trans. Biomed. Eng.* **2016,** *63* (3), 664–675. DOI: 10.1109/TBME.2015.2468589.
12. Krizhevsky, A.; Alex; Sutskever, I.; Hinton, G. E. Imagenet Classification with Deep Convolutional Neural Networks. *Adv. Neural Inf. Process. Syst.* **2012,** *25*, 1097–1105.
13. LeCun, Y.; Jackel, L. D.; Bottou, L.; Cortes, C.; Denker, J. S.; Drucker, H.; Guyon, I.; et al. Learning Algorithms for Classification: A Comparison on Handwritten Digit Recognition. *Neural Netw.: Stat. Mech. Perspect.* **1995** 261 (276), 2.
14. Li, S.; Wang, L.; Li, J.; Yao, Y. Image Classification Algorithm Based on Improved AlexNet. *J. Phys.: Conf. Ser.* **2021,** *1813*, 12051.
15. Li, X.; Yang, Y.; Pang, Zaihu; Wu, X. A Comparative Study on Selecting Acoustic Modeling Units in Deep Neural Networks Based Large Vocabulary Chinese Speech Recognition. *Neurocomputing* **2015,** *170*, 251–256. DOI: 10.1016/j.neucom.2014.07.087.
16. Liu, Y.; Chen, X.; Peng, H.; Wang, Z. Multi-Focus Image Fusion with a Deep Convolutional Neural Network. *Inf. Fusion* **2017,** *36*, 191–207. DOI: 10.1016/j.inffus.2016.12.001.
17. Majnaric, L.; Sabanovic, S. Cardiovascular Disease Research by Using Data from Electronic Health Records. *Atherosclerosis* **2016,** *252*, e41. DOI: 10.1016/j.atherosclerosis.2016.07.365.
18. Mashrur, F. R.; Dutta Roy, A. D.; Saha, D. K. Automatic Identification of Arrhythmia from ECG Using AlexNet Convolutional Neural Network. In *2019 4th International Conference on Electrical Information and Communication Technology (EICT)*; 2019; pp 1–5. DOI: 10.1109/EICT48899.2019.9068806.

19. Nannaparaju, V.; Narasimman, S. Detection of T-Wave Alternans in ECGs by Wavelet Analysis. *Proc. Mater. Sci.* **2015,** *10*, 307–313. DOI: 10.1016/j.mspro.2015.06.055.
20. Pandey, S. K.; Janghel, R. R. Automatic Detection of Arrhythmia from Imbalanced ECG Database Using CNN Model with SMOTE. *Australas. Phys. Eng. Sci. Med.* **2019,** *42* (4), 1129–1139. DOI: 10.1007/s13246-019-00815-9.
21. Prentašić, P.; Lončarić, S. Detection of Exudates in Fundus Photographs Using Deep Neural Networks and Anatomical Landmark Detection Fusion. *Comput. Methods Programs Biomed.* **2016,** *137*, 281–292. DOI: 10.1016/j.cmpb.2016.09.018.
22. Priya, K. D.; Rao, G. S.; Rao, P. S. V. S. Comparative Analysis of Wavelet Thresholding Techniques with Wavelet-Wiener Filter on ECG Signal. *Proc. Comput. Sci.* **2016,** *87*, 178–183. DOI: 10.1016/j.procs.2016.05.145.
23. Remya, R. S.; Indiradevi, K. P.; Babu, K. K. A. Classification of Myocardial Infarction Using Multi-Resolution Wavelet Analysis of ECG. *Proc. Technol.* **2016,** *24*, 949–956. DOI: 10.1016/j.protcy.2016.05.195.
24. Rhif, M.; Ben Abbes, A.; Farah, I. R.; Martínez, B.; Sang, Y. Wavelet Transform Application for/in Non-Stationary Time-Series Analysis: A Review. *Appl. Sci.* **2019,** *9* (7), 1345. DOI: 10.3390/app9071345
25. Sangaiah, A. K.; Arumugam, M.; Bian, G.-B. An Intelligent Learning Approach for Improving ECG Signal Classification and Arrhythmia Analysis. *Artif. Intell. Med.* **2020,** *103*, 101788. DOI: 10.1016/j.artmed.2019.101788.
26. Sannino, G.; De Pietro, G. A Deep Learning Approach for ECG-Based Heartbeat Classification for Arrhythmia Detection. *Fut. Gener. Comput. Syst.* **2018,** *86*, 446–455. DOI: 10.1016/j.future.2018.03.057.
27. Srivastava, N.; Hinton, G.; Krizhevsky, A.; Sutskever, I.; Salakhutdinov, R. Dropout: A Simple Way to Prevent Neural Networks from Overfitting. *J. Mach. Learn. Res.* **2014,** *15* (1), 1929–1958.
28. Tao, Q.; Zhan, S. Z.; Li, X.-H.; Kurihara, T. Robust Face Detection Using Local CNN and SVM Based on Kernel Combination. *Neurocomputing* **2016,** *211*, 98–105. DOI: 10.1016/j.neucom.2015.10.139.
29. Thomas, M.; Das, M. Kr.; Ari, S. Automatic ECG Arrhythmia Classification Using Dual-Tree Complex Wavelet Based Features. *A.E.U. Int. J. Electron. Commun.* **2015,** *69* (4), 715–721. DOI: 10.1016/j.aeue.2014.12.013.
30. Weimann; Kuba; Conrad, T. O. F. Transfer Learning for ECG Classification. *Sci. Rep.* **2021,** *11* (1), 1.
31. Yıldırım, Ö.; Pławiak, P.; Tan, R. S.; Acharya, U. R. Arrhythmia Detection Using Deep Convolutional Neural Network with Long Duration ECG Signals. *Comput. Biol. Med.* **2018,** *102*, 411–420. DOI: 10.1016/j.compbiomed.2018.09.009.
32. Yochum, M.; Renaud, C.; Jacquir, S. Automatic Detection of P, QRS and T Patterns in 12 Leads ECG Signal Based on CWT. *Biomed. Signal Process. Control* **2016,** *25*, 46–52. DOI: 10.1016/j.bspc.2015.10.011.

CHAPTER 14

MLO and CC View of Feature Fusion and Mammogram Classification Using a Deep Convolution Neural Network

V. SRIDEVI[1] and J. ABDUL SAMATH[2]

[1]*Department of Computer Science, PSG College of Arts & Science and Research Scholar of Government Arts College, Udumalpet, Tamil Nadu, India*

[2]*Department of Computer Science, Chikkanna Government Arts College, Tirupur, Tamil Nadu, India*

ABSTRACT

Breast cancer is a frequent type of cancer in women all over the world. The improvement of computer-aided system helps the radiologist with the effective analysis and diagnosis of breast cancer. It presents a computational methodology for classifying mammogram cancer as normal, benign, and malignant from the CC and MLO views of mammogram images. The proposed strategy consists of feature extraction, multiple-view feature fusion, and classification. The input images are fed into feature extraction where convolution neural network (CNN) is applied. The CNN is well suited for feature extraction, feature fusion, and mammogram classification. In this framework, the convolution layer, pooling, and activation function are used as feature extraction techniques. After the process of feature extraction, feature fusion is employed by the average pooling of CNN. The feature fusion will increase or maximize the relevant information of the breast image. Finally, obtained features from the fusion are fed into the CNN classifier, in which

Applied Intelligence for Medical Image Analysis. Aarti, Raju Pal, Mukesh Saraswat, & Himanshu Mittal (Eds.)

softmax and fully connected layers are employed as classifier techniques. The proposed work achieves 96.4% accuracy in classifying breast cancer from MLO and CC views using a hybrid feature with the CNN classifier.

14.1 INTRODUCTION

Breast cancer is found in women, and it causes a high mortality rate among them in India. In all countries, this type of disease is the main one in women.[1] Early identification of mammogram cancer has a higher chance of being cured. The global government, in collaboration with various health professionals, raises awareness about the risk of this disease among women. Therefore, early discovery is the perfect way to anticipate this infection. The most common early discovery of breast cancer is done through mammography, which provides a digital image of the breast. Through this, the clinical professional specialist distinguishes or visualizes the lesions or non-lesions in the breast.[2,3]

The radiologist missed some features at the time of visualization of breast cancer in mammogram, which led to a false diagnosis. This results in an error rate of 10–20% for malignant cancer.[4] The suspicious tissues are evacuated from the breast and given to a breast biopsy to test for the presence of breast cancer or not.[5]

A CAD system is used to analyze the medical image and offer reliable results. The CAD system assists the radiologist and lowers the number of false outcomes (Sridevi et al. 2010). With the help of a computer-based system, unnecessary biopsies are reduced by the computer-based diagnosis system, and the radiologist identifies breast cancer, which helps to decrease the mortality rate.

Many computer vision applications,[27,28] as well as applications linked to mammography analysis, such as mass segmentation,[26] mass detection,[28] and mammogram classification,[25] have given better results using deep learning models. Deep learning models' success is due to their ability to learn and incorporate all features by a series of hidden layers in the network structure.[31]

The research aim of this to build a deep convolution neural network (CNN) for assisting the radiologists in classifying mammography mass lesions and increasing the accuracy rate. This work has been carried out in MATLAB using CBIS-DDSM dataset.

The proposed framework is primarily based on two-view-based feature extraction and feature fusion techniques that are assessed on CBIS-DDSM mammogram images. In this chapter, the analysis of MLO and CC views is performed through the CAD method. The proposed system comprises three important phases of the CAD system: feature extraction, feature fusion of two view features, and mammogram classification. Two-view multiset of features are extracted using convolutional and pooling layers, which greatly increase the classification rate. Then multiple view features are concatenated and reduced by the feature fusion technique, which uses an average pooling method. Lastly, the fused features were input into the fully connected layer and the softmax classifier for classification of mammograms.

14.2 RELATED WORK

The suspicious region between the left and right mammograms is detected through structural variations between the two regions.[6]

de Sampaio et al.[8] developed a method for the detection of mass. In this method, the first tissue density is detected and classified the candidate region using SVM classifier. As a consequence, the sensitivity is 94.01%, the specificity is 82.25%, and the accuracy is 84.06% as a consequence.

Raghavendra et al.[10] extracted the features using Gabor Wavelet and selected the appropriate features or reduced them using the Locality Sensitive Discriminant Analysis method. Then, the resultant features are put into the K-NN classifier to classify the mammogram. They obtained an accuracy of 98.69%.

Khehra and Pharwaha[12] devised a hybrid technique for the mammogram cancer classification in which genetic algorithm and SVM techniques are applied. Dalalyan et al.[22] generated a hybrid method for the identification of mammogram cancer. In this approach, they used MIAS and the BCDR standard benchmark breast cancer dataset. Supervised techniques are employed in this method for the extraction of features. The resultant feature vectors are given in a hybrid method of SVM and DCNN classifier. They obtained a sensitivity of 98.75%. The drawback of this structure is its highly complex value network.

Ciecholewski[11] collected the mammogram images from DDSM and the MIAS database. They used contour approaches, including geometric active contour and active contour without edges, as well as the damping coefficient (EM) for the classifier. When the three types of contours are used, it causes a lack of microcalcifications.

Shankar and Ranjana (2018) developed an adaptive neuro-fuzzy inference system for mass enhancement and classification. They attained an accuracy of 98.91%. Rakhlin et al. (2018) used VGG, inception, and ResNet for the classification of mammogram images.

Berbar et al.[4] presented a method for classifying mammograms into mass and non-mass using three phases: image preprocessing, feature extraction, and classification. They proposed their method for the DDSM and MIAS databases and SVM used for classification. They extract the features using a hybrid method, which combines statistical features with texture features. The obtained feature vector is fed into the SVM classifier to classify it. They got 8.82% sensitivity and 98.69% specificity.

Prabhpreet et al. (2019) established a hybrid technique for breast cancer mammography image detection. The noise is first reduced by combining the work of the median and mean filters. This phase's output is fed into the K-mean clustering algorithm for feature extraction. To categorize the mammography picture into normal, the recovered feature vectors are fed into a multisupport vector machine.

Sridevi et al.[30] developed mammogram classification in which the suspicious region is segmented using the adaptive K-means segmentation algorithm and the KMC-GF feature extraction approach is used. K-NN classifier with KCM-GF feature extraction outperforms GLCM features for mammogram cancer.

14.3 METHODOLOGY

For the proposed methodology, the CBIS-DDSM dataset was used. Each image consists of a craniocaudal and a medio-lateral oblique view of the mammogram. A total of 2581 images were collected from the CBIS_DDSM cancer data set, of which 2197 are training images and 384 are testing images. The proposed framework consists of feature extraction, feature fusion, and classification. Figure 14.1 depicts the suggested architecture for breast cancer classification in its entirety.

Convolutional and pooling layers are used in feature extraction to extract features from each view of a mammography image. It extracts the multiple view features from the CC and MLO view mammogram images.

So, feature fusion is needed to merge the multiple features into a single vector. Finally, the given mammogram image is classified by the fully connected layer of CNN.

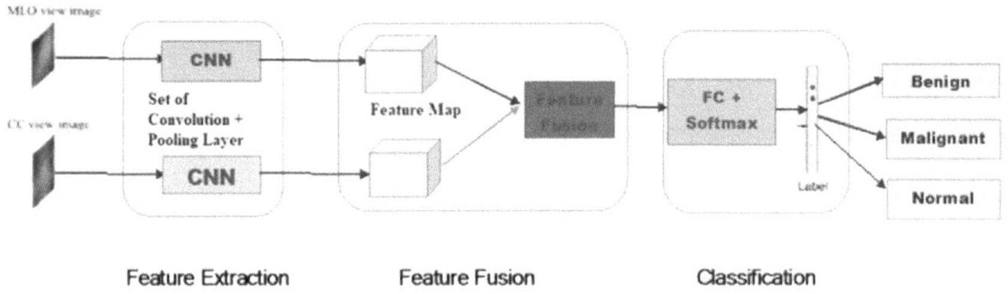

FIGURE 14.1 Architecture of breast cancer classification.

The proposed architecture of CNN with feature fusion employed CNN training for each mammographic view to discover masses in the image. To detect matching pairings of masses on the CC and MLO perspectives, the results of two CNNs are fused. Each CNN is divided into four sections, each of which has one convolution layer followed by a maxpooling layer. The convolutional layer is frequently referred to as a filter or a kernel that is convolved with the input as a set of weights. The filtering is carried out on a region-by-region basis. The activation function of the rectified linear unit (ReLU) is applied to the convolution layer to incorporate nonlinearities into the model via the resulting output map. The pooling layer separates the input image patch into a series of rectangles that do not overlap. Through the pooling layer, the number of parameters and the quantity of processing in the network can be minimized, allowing overlearning to be controlled.

The dataset is first divided into two sets for CNN training. In that, training set is training the network and the validation set is measuring the CNN training performance for each epoch. There were 150 epochs in the training procedure. We adjusted the initial learning rate to 0.0001 based on training performance.

The size of the RGB image of the input layer of the CNN architecture is $128 \times 128 \times 1$. The first convolutional layer's input dimension is $128 \times 128 \times 1$. In this case, each block consists of one convolutional layer with 16 channels and 2×2 maxpooling layer with stride 2×2. The resultant feature map is $8 \times 8 \times 128$ pixels at last. After the fourth block of CNN training, we add a feature fusion layer average pooling of CNN to create our modified model. A feature fusion layer was added to create a 4 × 4 × 128 feature vector. The output of a feature fusion layer is a 4 × 4 × 128 feature vector. The end layer is FC with the feature fusion. It's commonly referred to as a decision layer. The classification vector acquired from FC is normalized using a softmax activation function at the end. In this framework, loss function is used. For each of the three classes, the FC layer outputs three channels. The normal output category is 0, the benign output category is 1, and the malignant output category is 2.

14.3.1 FEATURE EXTRACTION

Through feature extraction, the relative features of mammogram images are obtained. In this proposed framework, a CNN is employed. During feature extraction, the number of convolution layers is changed. For each view, four convolutional layers and four maximum pooling layers are exercised to extract the features. To discover where the neurons' output is related to the input local areas, the convolution layer calculates the scalar product between the input and weights. The goal of the pooling layer is to lower the input's spatial dimensionality and the number of parameters in the activation. The feature extraction is evaluated using an activation function such as ReLU. The activation of ReLU is

$$f(x) = \begin{cases} 0 & for \quad x < 0 \\ x & for \quad x \geq 0 \end{cases}$$

A CNN is effective in image classification problems due to the spatially correlated features of the image given by convolution operation. Convolution is obtained by initialization of a square matrix with specific values. The obtained matrix is applied to each pixel of the mammogram image. A maximum pooling layer follows the convolution layer.

To construct the convolution layer's entire output volume, each kernel in a CNN has an activation map which is stacked with the depth dimension. By improving the model's output, the convolution layer helps to reduce the model's complexity. These optimizations for depth, stride, and zero-padding are used. The convolution layer generates the output volume depth based on a controlled setup of the number of neurons inside the layer at the same input region. To specify the stride, set the depth around the input's spatial dimensions. The border of the input is padded using the zero-padding method.

Each convolutional neural network employs four convolutional layers for extracting features. Each convolutional layer has convolutional kernels with 1 stride and max pooling layer with 2 stride. A concatenation layer is used at the network's end to integrate the generated feature maps. The input is 128 × 128 pixels in size.

The convolution layer takes a 2D matrix. The single output matrix of the convolution layer is given by the below equation:

$$C_j = f\left(\sum_{i=1}^{N} \tilde{M}_i * K_{i,j} + B_j\right)$$

where $\tilde{M}_i$ represent the input matrix which convolves with the kernel matrix $K_{i,j}$, B_j represents the bias that is added to the output after the sum of all convoluted matrix is computed, f represents the nonlinear activation function.

14.3.2 FEATURE FUSION

The research aim is to propose two-view feature fusion network model to fully exploit the complementary relationship between the two perspectives. As a result, average pooling is used in this framework to minimize the number of features from each patient's two mammography scans. We employed the global average operation at this point to reduce the picture feature to a one-dimensional vector, which was then given into the fully connected layer of the network. This feature fusion approach significantly increases the system performance. This method's purpose is to lower the prediction error. We stack the two views' feature vectors and they are represented as

$$Z_v = \left\lfloor z^{(1)};\ldots; z^{(ny)} \right\rfloor \in R^{1\times D\times ny}$$

and applying average-pooling across them is shown in the above equation.

14.3.3 MAMMOGRAM CLASSIFICATION

The classification attempts to classify the mammograms. In this step, the fused features are given into a fully connected layer, which is subsequently passed on to the softmax classifier. The number of output classes in the softmax classifier is the number of outputs. To connect our proposed architecture, we used nonlinear protocol tan *h*. The softmax function is a squashing function that re-normalizes the k-dimensional input vector, yielding a range of real values between Ferlay et al.[1] and Junior et al.[2] It can be expressed mathematically as

$$\sigma(z)_j = \frac{e^{zj}}{\sum_{k=1}^{K} e^{zk}}, \ for \ j = 1, \ldots K$$

Overfitting and underfitting phenomena frequently impair deep learning training. We used batch normalization after each layer in our proposed architecture to address these concerns. After the first fully connected layer, the dropout was added.

14.3.4 LOSS FUNCTION

The adjusting of loss function and upgrading the network design improved the performance of classification. The weighted loss function was

$$L(w, x_i, y_i) = -\frac{1}{N}\sum_{j=1}^{k} t_{ji} \ln y_{jn}$$

Here, x_i is the input vector, y_i is the classifier's prediction for the *n*th clinical input data, and t_n is the *n*th clinical sample's actual response. The number of classes is *K*, while *N* is the total number of samples.

14.4 RESULT AND DISCUSSION

We test our method on a dataset: CBIS-DDSM. The assessment datasets, the experimental setting, and the specifics of our approach's experimental implementation are presented first in this work. Our method's experimental findings are then thoroughly examined.

14.4.1 DATA SET

The CBIS-DDSM is used to train and assess the model. In this part, a total of 5162 samples were taken from 2581 breasts. Based on radiologists' diagnoses, we retrieved 1018 normal, 766 benign, and 797 malignant breasts.

All of the data is separated into two categories: training and testing. There are 890 normal breasts, 638 benign, and 669 malignant mammograms in the training set. There are 128 normal breasts, 128 benign, and 128 malignant mammograms in the testing set. We proportionally partition the training data into 10 subsets so that we may test the model's performance using 10-fold cross-validation. Table 14.1 represents the composition of the dataset used for the experimentation. Figure 14.2 depicts the visualization of each class of mammogram image.

TABLE 14.1 Composition of Dataset Used for the Experimentation.

Type	Normal	Benign	Malignant	Total
Train	890	638	669	2197
Test	128	128	128	384
Total	1018	766	797	2581

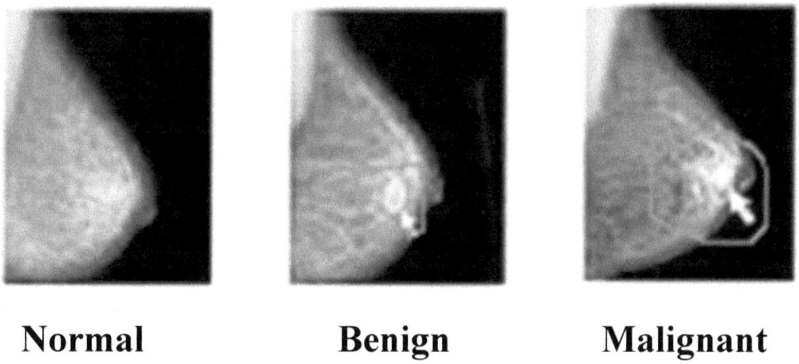

FIGURE 14.2 Visualization of each class of mammogram.

14.4.2 EXPERIMENTAL SETUP

Modern CNNs are frequently constructed by series of convolutional layers on top of the input, then connecting the classification output with FC layers. The improving of translational invariance and reducing the feature map size was done by max pooling layers. In each block, a convolution filter of the same depth is followed by a max pooling layer of stride 2 that shrinks the feature map by a factor of two. Table 14.1 shows the network architecture of our coding system in detail. It is possible to converge after 100 epochs, as indicated in Table 14.2. Finally, we employed ReLU as an activation function for each convolutional layer. Aside from that, batch normalization was used to speed up deep network training.

TABLE 14.2 Network Architecture of Proposed System.

Type	Kernel with stride	Output size
Convol1	3 × 3 × 16	128 × 128 × 16
Pool1	2 × 2 × 2	64 × 64 × 16
Convol2	3 × 3 × 32	64 × 64 × 31
Pool2	2 × 2 × 2	32 × 32 × 32
Convol3	3 × 3 × 64	32 × 32 × 64
Pool3	2 × 2 × 2	16 × 16 × 64
Convol4	3 × 3 × 128	16 × 16 × 128
Pool4	2 × 2 × 2	8 × 8 × 128
Feature fusion	2 × 2 × 2	4 × 4 × 128
Fully connected		1 × 1 × 64
Softmax		1 × 1 × 64

14.4.3 PERFORMANCE METRICS

The feature fusion with the CNN system's performance allows it to correctly classify standard medical metrics are used to evaluate mammograms at all stages. They are sensitivity, specificity, F1 score, and accuracy. Sensitivity refers to the ability of a model to anticipate the positive outcome of a test. When the actual test is also positive, a mammogram is recommended. The term "specificity" refers to a model's ability to predict the negative class. The confusion matrix from the classifier output is used to evaluate the proposed system's performance measures.

$$Accuracy = (TP + TN) / (TN + TP + TP + FN)$$

$$Sentitivity = TP / (TP + FN)$$

$$Specificity = TN / (TN + FP)$$

$$F1\ Score = (2 * TP) / (2 * TP + FP + FN)$$

$$AUC = \frac{sensitivity + Specificity}{2}$$

where TP is the exactly classified abnormal cases as abnormal; FP is the incorrectly classified normal cases as abnormal; TN is the exactly classified normal cases as normal; and FN is the incorrectly classified abnormal cases as normal.

14.4.4 RESULT ANALYSIS

We used CNN architecture and multiple view feature fusion with CNN techniques to investigate and measure network performance. Table 14.3 shows the outcomes of putting the various network topologies to the test.

TABLE 14.3 Comparative Performance of CNN without Fusion and Feature Fusion with CNN.

Method	Accuracy (%)	Sensitivity (%)	Specificity (%)	F1 score (%)
CNN without fusion	92.2	93.5	92.8	94.4
Feature fusion with CNN (proposed method)	96.4	96.3	–95.2	94.9

The feature fusion with the CNN classifier provides a better recognition rate compared to CNN without fusion. The feature fusion with the CNN classifier has the advantage of texture and neural network specification features. Positive and negative likelihood are used to test the ability to predict positive and negative classes on a confusion matrix. For a more thorough analysis of the proposed system, we used the ROC curve and the area under the ROC to evaluate our models. The ROC plot is a two-dimensional space with the x-axis representing the false-positive rate (one specificity) and the y-axis representing the true positive rate of the system (sensitivity). The assessment of accuracy was done by area under the ROC.

As shown in Figure 14.3, the area under the ROC curve (AUC) for the CNN and feature fusion with CNN designs was calculated to be 97.9%

and 95.2%, respectively, clearly demonstrating that the suggested network outperformed the CNN architecture.

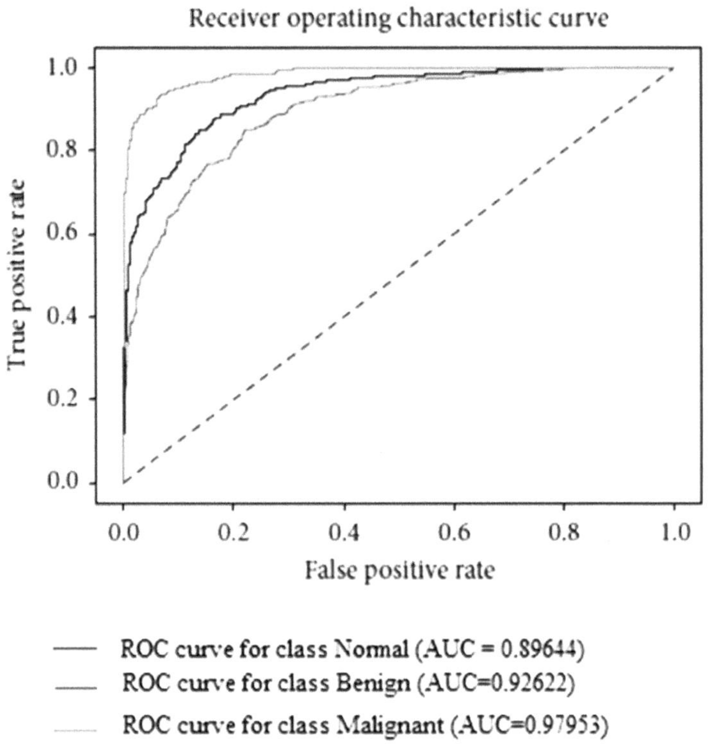

FIGURE 14.3 ROC curve of the average performance using fusion after reduction approach.

14.4.5 COMPARISON WITH STATE-OF-THE-ART MAMMOGRAM CLASSIFICATION

Table 14.4 compares the performance of our method with other deep learning-based methods. Sun et al.[32] developed a novel architecture that extracts features from two views of the breast mass. The model included dilated convolutional layers that fused the features from the multiple breast masses. In addition, they included a penalty component in loss function, which allows the model to minimize the misclassification rate.

Yang et al.[33] presented tri-view mass identification approach based on DNN that can analyze mammographic pictures bilaterally and ipsilaterally at the same time, emulating radiologists' reading practice. The symmetry and geometry constraints are learned by high-resolution network architectures and concatenated the features from all views.

Shu et al.[34] suggested a deep neural network-based full mammography classification algorithm. The two structures' region and global max pooling were used to handle the challenge of classifying tiny lesions in the entire mammogram. They implemented the proposed two pooling structures on a fine-trained AlexNet network for classification.

Table 14.4 clearly shows that the accuracy of our proposed system, which is a two-view fused deep convolutional feature, was higher than single-view deep convolutional feature. The optimal performance indicated the algorithm effectiveness and it proved with the aid of testing and performance analysis.

TABLE 14.4 Comparison of Mammogram Classification with Other.

Method	Data set	Accuracy (%)	Sensitivity (%)	AUC (%)
Sun et al.[32]	DDSM and MIAS	82.02	–	–
Yang et al.[33]	DDSM	96.2	89.92	91.44
Shu et al.[34]	CBIS-DDSM	92.2	–	92.4
Our proposed	CBIS-DDSM	96.4	96.3	94.9

14.5 CONCLUSION

Two views are used in this framework: the MLO and CC view models. The information retrieved from these perspectives is utilized to classify them. The proposed two views of MLO and CC normal and abnormal models provide a greater recognition rate than single-view-based system. The experimental results suggest that by employing a two-view feature extraction and feature fusion system, the proposed method improves. Furthermore, a comparison analysis demonstrates that the proposed designs outperform other mammography classification systems significantly. The suggested effort will aid in the detection of MLO and CC views of mammogram cancer.

KEYWORDS

- **mammogram**
- **breast cancer**
- **convolution neural network (CNN)**
- **feature extraction**
- **feature fusion**
- **convolution**
- **pooling**
- **MLO and CC views**
- **classification**

REFERENCES

1. Ferlay, J.; Soerjomataram, I.; Dikshit, R.; Eser, S.; Mathers, C.; Rebelo, M.; Parkin, D. M.; Forman, D.; Bray, F. Cancer Incidence and Mortality Worldwide: Sources, Methods and Major Patterns in Globocan 2012. *Int. J. Cancer* **2015,** *136* (5), E359–E386. DOI: 10.1002/ijc.29210.
2. Junior, G. B.; da Rocha, S. V.; Gattass, M.; Silva, A. C.; de Paiva, A. C. A Mass Classification Using Spatial Diversity Approaches in Mammography Images for False Positive Reduction. *Expert Syst. Appl.* **2013,** *40* (18), 7534–7543.
3. Sampaio, W. B.; Diniz, E. M.; Silva, A. C.; De Paiva, A. C.; Gattass, M. Detection of Masses in Mammogram Images Using CNN, Geostatistic Functions and SVM. *Comput. Biol. Med.* **2011,** *41* (8), 653–664. DOI: 10.1016/j.compbiomed.2011.05.017.
4. Berbar, M. A. Hybrid Methods for Feature Extraction for Breast Masses Classification. *Egypt. Inform. J.* **2018,** *19*, 63–73.
5. Thawkar, S.; Ingolikar, R. Classification of Masses in Digital Mammograms Using Biogeography-Based Optimization Technique. *J. King Saud Univ. Comput. Inf. Sci.* **2020,** *32* (10), 1140–1148.
6. Ericeira, D.R.; Silva, A. C.; De Paiva, A. C.; Gattass, M. Detection of Masses Based on Asymmetric Regions of Digital Bilateral Mammograms Using Spatial Description with Variogram and Cross-Variogram Functions. *Comput. Biol. Med.* **2013,** *43* (8), 987–999.
7. Kaur, P.; Singh, G.; Kaur, P. Intellectual Detection and Validation of Automated Mammogram Breast Cancer Images by Multi-Class SVM Using Deep Learning Classification. *Inform. Med. Unlocked* **2019,** *16*, 100151.
8. de Sampaio, B.; Silva, A. C.; de Paiva, A. C.; Gattass, M. Detection of Masses in Mammograms with Adaption to Breast Density Using Genetic Algorithm, Phylo-Genetic Trees, LBP and SVM. *Expert Syst. Appl.* **2015,** *42* (22), 8911–8928.

9. Abdel-Nasser, M.; Moreno, A.; Puig, D. Temporal Mammogram Image Registration Using Optimized Curvilinear Coordinates. *Comput. Methods Programs Biomed.* **2016,** *127*, 1–14. DOI: 10.1016/j.cmpb.2016.01.019.
10. Raghavendra, U.; Acharya, R. U.; Fujita, H.; Gudigar, A. Tan, J.H.; Chokkadi, S. Application of Gabor Wavelet and Locality Sensitive Discriminant Analysis for Automated Identification of Breast Cancer Using Digitized Mammogram Images. *Appl. Soft Comput. J.* **2016,** *46*, 151–161.
11. Ciecholewski, M. Malignant and Benign Mass Segmentation in Mammograms Using Active Contour Methods. *Symmetry* **2017,** *9* (11), 1–22. DOI: 10.3390/sym9110277.
12. Khehra, B. S.; Pharwaha, A. P. S. Comparison of Genetic Algorithm, Particle Swarm Optimization and Biogeography-Based Optimization for Feature Selection to Classify Clusters of Microcalcifications. *J. Inst. Eng. India. Ser. B*: *India Ser.* **2017,** *98* (2), 189–202. DOI: 10.1007/s40031-016-0226-8.
13. Haralick, R. M.; Shanmugam, K.; Dinstein, I. Textural Features for Image Classification. *IEEE Trans. Syst. Man Cybern.* **1973,** *6* (6), 610–621. DOI: 10.1109/TSMC.1973.4309314.
14. Duraisamy, S.; Emperumal, S. Computer-Aided Mammogram Diagnosis System Using Deep Learning Convolutional Fully Complex-Valued Relaxation Neural Network Classifier. *Deep Learn. Comput. Vis.* **2017,** *11* (8), 656–662.
15. Campilho, A.; Karray, F.; ter Haar Romeny, B., Eds. Image Analysis and Recognition. In *ICIAR 2018. Lecture Notes in Computer Science*; Springer: Chamdoi, 2018; Vol. 10882.
16. Johnson, J. L.; Ritter, D. Observation of Periodic Waves in a Pulse-Coupled Neural Network. *Opt. Lett.* **1993,** *18* (15), 1253–1255. DOI: 10.1364/ol.18.001253.
17. Ranganath, H. S.; Kuntimad, G.; Johnson, J. L. Pulse Coupled Neural Networks for Image Processing. In *Proc. of the Southeast Conference on 'Visualize the future'*; 1995; pp 37–43.
18. Wang, Z.; Ma, Y.; Cheng, F.; Yang, L. Review of Pulse-Coupled Neural Networks. *Image Vis. Comput.* **2010,** *28* (1), 5–13. DOI: 10.1016/j.imavis.2009.06.007.
19. O'Shea, K.; Nash, R. An Introduction to Convolutional Neural Networks.. *ArXiv e* **2015**. ArXiv e-Prints.
20. Albawi, S.; Mohammed, T. A.; Alzawi, S. Understanding of a Convolutional Neural Network. In *International Conference on Engineering and Technology (ICE T)*; 2017. DOI: 10.1109/ICENGTECHNOL.2017.8308186.
21. Wu, J. *Convolutional Neural Networks*; LAMDA Group, National Key Laboratory for Novel Software Technology, Nanjing University: Nanjing, 2020.
22. Jouirou, A.; Baâzaoui, A.; Barhoumi, W. Multi-View Information Fusion in Mammograms: A Comprehensive Overview. *Inf. Fusion* **2019,** *52*, 308–321_321. DOI: 10.1016/j.inffus.2019.05.001.
23. Sridevi, V.; Abdul Samath, J. A Survey on Breast Cancer Segmentation and Classification Using Several Methods. *Int. J. Sci. Res. Comput. Sci. Appl. Manage. Stud.* **2019,** *8* (3).
24. Carneiro, G.; Nascimento, J.; Bradley, A. P. *Unregistered Multiview Mammogram Analysis with Pretrained Deep Learning Models, MICCAI*; Springer: Cham, 2015; pp 652–660.

25. Dhungel, N.; Carneiro, G.; Bradley, A. P. *Deep Learning and Structured Prediction for the Segmentation of Mass in Mammograms, MICCAI*; Springer: Cham, 2015; pp 605–612.
26. Krizhevsky, A.; Sutskever, I.; Hinton, G. E. Imagenet Classification with Deep Convolutional Neural Networks. *NIPS* **2012,** *1*, 4.
27. He, K.; Zhang, X.; Ren, S.; Sun, J. Deep Residual Learning for Image Recognition. *arXiv* **2015**. arXiv:1512.03385.
28. Carneiro, N. D. G.; Bradley, A. P. *Automated Mass Detection in Mammograms Using Cascaded Deep Learning and Random Forests, DICTA*; IEEE: New York, NY, 2015; pp 1–8.
29. Sridevi, V.; Abdul Samath, J. Advancement on Breast Cancer Detection Using Medio-Lateral-Oblique (MLO) and Cranio-Caudal (CC) Features. *Test Eng. Manage.* **2020,** *83* (May–June), 85–93.
30. Szegedy, C.; Liu, W.; Jia, Y.; Sermanet, P.; Reed, S.; Anguelov, D.; Erhan, D.; Vanhoucke, V.; Rabinovich, A.; Vanhoucke, V.; Rabinovich, A. Going Deeper with Convolutions. In *IEEE Conference on Computer Vision and Pattern Recognition (CVPR)*; 2015; pp 1–9. DOI: 10.1109/CVPR.2015.7298594.
31. Sun, L.; Wang, J.; Hu, Z.; Xu, Y.; Cui, Z. Multi-View Convolutional Neural Networks for Mammographic Image Classification. *IEEE Access* **2019,** *7*, 126273–126282. DOI: 10.1109/ACCESS.2019.2939167.
32. Yang, Z.; Cao, Z.; Zhang, Y.; Tang, Y.; Lin, X.; Ouyang, R.; Wu, M.; Han, M.; Xiao, J.; Huang, L.; Wu, S.; Chang, P.; Ma, J. MommiNet v. Mammographic Multi-view Mass Identification Networks. *Med. Image Anal.* **2021,** *73*, 102204. ISSN: 1361-8415. DOI: 10.1016/j.media.2021.102204.
33. Shu, X.; Zhang, L.; Wang, Z.; Lv, Q.; Yi, Z. Deep Neural Networks with Region-Based Pooling Structures for Mammographic Image Classification. *IEEE Trans. Med. Imaging* **2020,** 39 (6), 2246–2255. DOI: 10.1109/TMI.2020.2968397.

Index

B

C

G

H

I

K

L

M

N